What Others Are Saying

Been in the fragrance retail world for twenty years and didn't know your blood type affected your fragrance scent. Deb is amazingly on target with this system. After working with her for over three years, I'm a believer!

—Sandy Duvall, Belk Estée Lauder Counter Manager

Deb has helped me find fragrance for my daughter in law…We talked about her personality and found what she thought would be a match based on her theory! Turned out that it did!

—Kim Medlin, Belk Customer

Deb has defined the relationship of fragrance, individuality, and human body chemistry. She has explained specific fragrances best suited for each person and why. Her extensive knowledge of scents will help you select the very best fragrance. This is a must-have book for anyone who uses fragrance or wishes to purchase a fine fragrance for themselves or for their loved ones.

—George and Mary Beth Pail, Belk Customers

Scent-Sational Searches

Scent-Sational Searches

Find Your Fragrance By Blood & Personality Parallels

Deborah Worley

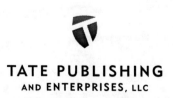

TATE PUBLISHING
AND ENTERPRISES, LLC

Published by Tate Publishing & Enterprises, LLC
127 E. Trade Center Terrace | Mustang, Oklahoma 73064 USA
1.888.361.9473 | www.tatepublishing.com

Tate Publishing is committed to excellence in the publishing industry. The company reflects the philosophy established by the founders, based on Psalm 68:11,
"The Lord gave the word and great was the company of those who published it."

Book design copyright © 2016 by Tate Publishing, LLC. All rights reserved.
Cover design by Jim Villaflores
Interior design by Jomar Ouano

Published in the United States of America

ISBN: 978-1-68118-535-4
1. Reference / General
2. Reference / Personal & Practical Guides
16.04.06

Dedicated to the memory of my dearest friend, Sandra Graham, who believed in me and my theory. Without her encouragement and enthusiasm, *Scent-sational Searches* would have never been published.

Perfume...is bottled emotion
that can reunite us with the past...
reminding us of what we once held close.

—*Good Housekeeping*, November 2011

Contents

Prologue
The "Fragranista" Begins

Hello, and thanks for your interest in *Scent-sational Searches*. I suppose my journey began when I was a mere child. I would always notice a wonderful distinctive difference about my daddy when he put on "Smell Good," as he referred to his Old Spice cologne. My mother wore her "Estée" (Estée Lauder perfume) for as long as I can remember. Her mother would sparingly dab on a bit of lavender for special occasions. These scents all evoke happy memories of family, and I'm sure they are the basis of my love for perfume.

My true passion began to unfold back in 2007 when I took a part-time job with Belk in Savannah, Georgia, as a fragrance consultant and sales representative. My adventure into the world of perfume definitely developed me into what I jokingly refer to today as a "fragranista"!

Soon after I began my job, I noticed a parallel among certain people and their fragrance choices. I was totally in the dark about the commonalities of who liked and bought what; however, my job description directed me to assist people with their fragrance selections.

Inquiring Mind

I often wondered why certain women would lean into a fragrance card or spray mist into the air then vocalize their delight with "oohhs" and "aahhs," while others would wrinkle their nose, frown, turn away from the aroma, and literally groan, "Eeeww! No! Not me!"

This inquiring mind also wanted to know why the same lovely perfume would seem to smell quite different on some people. I began a search to discover more and more about fragrance notes and their families. I learned how to describe perfume to my customers as if the beautifully bottled concoctions were fine wines from which they could choose a favorite!

After a while I realized that I was definitely on to something big! And so, my curiosity began to beautifully blossom, as did my joy and exhilaration of this quest for more knowledge about the mystery that now unfolded before me.

Observations

While working in Savannah, my first observations indicated that many women of color (predominantly O blood types) seemed to love the traditional heavier scents of flowers with woodsy or spicy notes. Japanese art students (predominantly A blood types) favored brighter mixed bouquets of fruity florals.

Other distinctive pieces of this puzzle were the obviously outdoorsy or athletic people who came into the store wearing their gym clothes or their golf or tennis attire. This group went for the more modern crisp green notes with citrus and cedars.

The fourth group I profiled as more quiet or sensitive. They tended to be a bit standoffish or indecisive and proved to be very difficult to assist. They navigated toward a slim fragrance selection of soft, clean smells that often dry down to a delicate powdery scent.

Patterns Begin

While searching for answers, I checked to see what, if anything, Stanford University might have published on this subject. The only thing relative that I could find was their introduction about *Ethnicity and Human Genetic Linkage Maps.* I learned that we are all born with genetic markers determined by our blood types. These genetic markers are the linkage maps that determine our physical traits—hair, eyes, skin color, height, etc.

Definite patterns began to materialize as I helped women and men search for the perfect perfumes that satisfied their senses. Their choices seemed to fall into categories that reflected an obvious personality or presumed blood type (the thing people kept referring to as body chemistry).

So I began to think that not only are these "markers" external, but they are also internal and that our body chemistry has much more than meets the eye. I believe that it also meets the nose, and my reality is that the nose truly does know!

Looking back on my own personal experiences, I suffered a serious lung disorder years ago. During my illness, one of the physicians from the Atlanta Center for Disease Control (CDC) turned me on to the book *Eat Right 4 Your Type.* This book by Dr. Peter D'Adamo is about how to eat based on your blood type. It has become an international bestseller.[1]

His book contends the following arguments:

Blood Type O thrives on a lean, high protein diet.

Blood Type A thrives on a primarily vegetarian diet.

Blood Type B thrives on a mixed diet of meat, fish, and dairy.

Blood Type AB thrives on a modified vegetarian diet.

Blood Studies

My life's experience in the medical arena had taught me that a person's body chemistry definitely determined the effect of certain foods *and* drugs that were ingested. Some were good, and others were not so much.

I decided that the same must surely be true about the use of fragrances and other scents. It's another facet of chemistry! So I decided to learn more about how our bodies respond to what we spray and rub into it and what, if any, was its correlation to blood types.

My studies showed that O is the blood type that claims the largest percentage of the population, with 44 percent in the USA having this type. Next is the A family, which makes up about 42 percent of the blood population in this country. These people were meat-eating "warriors" and "hunters."

After man became "farmers," the next two blood types evolved. The B group came next, and presently, it represents less than 12 percent of the blood population. It was followed by the AB type at about 4 percent. The AB type evolved only about five hundred years ago. This group is extremely sensitive and is more prone to illness.[2]

Personality Parallels

I began to truly believe that individual body chemistry (blood type) and personality type did in fact have correlated factors that absolutely influenced fragrance choices. So I began a search to confirm my theory about such parallels.

My research led to Japanese studies that began back in the 1920s to determine which blood type would produce the best soldiers. Not surprisingly, a parallel between blood types and personality types was indicated.

It pointed to the Bs as the best soldiers. Their personality can be aggressive and competitive. I have also noticed that these folks play to win. Second place just does not count! Also, the Os made the best officers. They are natural leaders with strong, decisive opinions.

That research died down in the 1940s, but it was revitalized in the 1970s. Today, this belief is a huge part of Japanese culture. (Read more about blood type parallels to personalities in chapter 2.)

Game On

My passion to prove what I called my fragranista theory led me to develop my own simple guessing game. I'd invite customers to "spray and play." If they had no clue about blood type, we'd talk about personalities to help determine a probable fragrance family choice, and I'd guide them in that direction. We did this instead of walking around the fragrance counters and trying bottle after bottle in the hope of finding something special that they liked.

My decisions about which fragrances worked best for which specific blood and personality types (B/PTs) began to come into focus. So I developed a brief survey that tied the two together and used it as a tool to confirm my beliefs about the correlation of B/PTs and fragrance choices.

The surveys revealed an accuracy rate of 80 to 90 percent and provided great documentation for my fragrance theory. Of course, there were always untypical responses, but my work became much easier and sales soared!

I advised customers to never buy a fragrance unless they absolutely loved it.

"Don't wear it because it smells good on a friend or relative. Chances are, it could smell totally different on you."

"And why is this?"

"Because of your body chemistry or blood type," I'd respond.

So it was "game on" for me! I absolutely loved the challenge!

Customer Comments

Over the years, customers' comments made their frustration to find a perfect perfume quite evident. Whether shopping in a brick-and-mortar store or searching online, it was not uncommon for people to become quite overwhelmed by literally tens of thousands of choices—from perfumes, lotions and soaps to candles, diffusers, and spray air fresheners. Not to mention what an expensive mistake is made when a fragrance purchase turns out to be not so good.

Repeatedly, I would hear, "I tried it [a fragrance] on the tester card [or sprayed it on] and thought I liked it. But after I bought it and took it home, I realized that it did not work for me at all!" Or, "It changes on me. It doesn't stay on me. It smells different on me than it does on my girlfriend. My hubby hates it!"

And my favorite:

"It smells just like bug spray on me!"

Fragrance 101

During my seven years of working in and researching the world of fragrance, I really enjoyed assisting customers with what I jokingly called "Fragrance 101." This truly empowered them to make an informed decision and to buy with confidence.

The encouragement of many customers, friends, and family prompted my decision to write this collection of my findings. I have tried diligently to give credit and reference where credit is due.

Scent-sational Searches is written for the person who just wants to know more about fragrances and how to be better able to find their perfect scents. It is filled with my research articles, personal observation, and opinions about fragrances. I pieced together this body of information that helped me to build and confirm my theory.

You will also find a great historical review from ancient to modern times. A chapter with one hundred Q and A facts is included. Plus, there are brief biographies of my four fave perfumers: Coco Chanel, Estée Lauder, Thierry Mugler, and Michael Edwards (the creator of the fragrance wheel). They have each spawned major changes that continue to influence the world of fragrance.

So enjoy! Armed with *Scent-sational Searches*, may you have a happy hunting for the perfect fragrances that you (and others) will truly love!

Scent-sationally yours,
Deborah Worley

1

Perfume Evolution

We begin with a brief history of how the perfume world evolved, beginning with European days of antiquity up to our modern-day industry. This chapter comes directly from one of my favorite reference sites, OsMoz.com., which is a social network for fragrance consumers. Its purpose is to allow access to opinions and advice from other consumers and to the expertise of Fimenich, the publisher of the site since 2001.

It is a member of an international association, The Fragrance Foundation. It was established in 1949 by six industry leaders affiliated with Elizabeth Arden, Coty, Guerlain, Helena Rubinstein, Chanel, and Parfums Weil to develop educational programs about the importance and pleasures of fragrance for the American public.

Today, America is the largest fragrance market in the world, and The Fragrance Foundation has become an international source for historic, cultural, scientific, and industry-related reference materials.

This is a wonderful site to explore and learn about fragrances for men and women. I find it to be one of the most interesting and informative sites online today.

The History of Fragrances

Perfume, as we know it today, began centuries ago on the borders of civilization and has created its own history. Its societal past indicates that it was used as "a means of exchange, a protection against disease, a potion with divine virtues."[1]

Antiquity

In early civilizations, from Egypt to Greece, fragrance did not exist as such. Scented flowers, plants, and other raw materials were dedicated as perfumed offerings to the gods.

As the years went by, interest in fragrant substances grew among both the rich and the poor. They began to utilize them increasingly in oils, balms, fumigations, and in fermented liquors in an effort to get closer to the gods. It was believed that fragrances could help perfect their bodies and give them healing power. However, during the years of decadence that followed this, high perceptions began to fall.

Middle Ages

During the Middle Ages, plants were used to protect against epidemics whereas perfumes from the orient whispered of carnal pleasures. The church condemned alchemists.[2]

Exploring crusaders brought new raw materials and fragrance techniques back from the Orient. European alchemists discovered ethyl alcohol and distillation from the Chinese and the Arabs. People believed that pleasant smells had disinfectant qualities and could protect against epidemics.

Marco Polo's travels gave tremendous boost to the spice trade. "Fragrance balls" carried around by the wealthy were filled with aromatic resins, amber, or musk to hide or ward off unpleasant smells.

> The use of fragrance ushered in a new art of living. Poets celebrated femininity with passion. In spite of a stern warning from the Church, the gentlemen and their ladies used sensual, scented baths to indulge in carnal pleasures. [3]

Renaissance 1490–1600

During the Renaissance period, a new vision of the world was ushered in. Progressive chemists began to replace the outdated perfume recipes of alchemists.

Architects, engineers, artists, and scholars traveled all over Europe. Vasco de Gama, Christopher Columbus, and Magellan were all famous explorers who brought back new raw materials from America and India. These included cocoa, vanilla, Peru balsam, tobacco, pepper, clove, and cardamom.

Foreign perfumers from Spain and Italy left their native countries to set up shop in Paris and to serve wealthy patrons. Famous courtesans, influential women, and even queens fought over secret formulas created by the first Italian chemists.

Classic Era 1600–1700

This era saw fragrance utilized to intoxicating levels at the Versailles court, which dictated fashion and customs. Instead of bathing, men and women used excessive amounts of fragrance and cosmetics.

Makers of gloves, fragrances, and powders became organized and developed their trade. The flowers of carnation, violet, jasmine, rose, tuberose, and lavender were in great demand. Perfumed gloves were sold all over France as a sign of fashion.

Century of Lights 1700–1789

> Hairstyles, make-up and perfume … During that era, women painstakingly followed the codes of seduction and discovered the tyranny of fashion. [4]

This century became a carefree time of celebration during the reign of Louis XV with Marie-Antoinette as its fashion focus. The "perfumed court" made hygiene fashionable once again, and different fragrances were often used.

As the olfactive taste evolved, more subtle fragrances were embraced. The first famous Parisian fragrance houses grew wealthy. The Grasse chemists had succeeded in improving the techniques of distillation. In Cologne, Jean-Antoine Farina launched the "eau de cologne."

Napoleonic Years 1789–1860

After the French Revolution, the flower-like women of this romantic era lost interest in makeup and strong fragrances. They sought delicate scents that reflected their personalities and pale faces. They were known to carry scented handkerchiefs in their hand.

British hygienists revived the popularity of fragrant baths. Empress Josephine spent freely on exotic scents while Napoleon enjoyed his addiction to body rubs with eau de cologne.

Modern Perfumery 1860–1900

Toward the end of the nineteenth century, a stronger middle class emerged. The perfume industry began to target these women who displayed a more refined taste in fragrance, and the excessive infatuation with vetiver and patchouli came to an end.

The birth of modern perfumery began with an olfactory revolution and the brand-new process of chemical synthesis. The first synthetic fragrance notes such as coumarin, vanillin, heliotropine, ionone, and the first aldehydes were created and introduced into fragrances. Perfumery became viewed more often as an art.

The Twentieth Century

Traditional Perfumery Emerges

The traditional classification which emerged around 1900 comprised the following categories:

- Single Floral: Fragrances that are dominated by a scent from one particular flower; in French called a soliflore. (e.g. Serge Lutens' Sa Majeste La Rose, which is dominated by rose.)
- Floral Bouquet: Is a combination of fragrance of several flowers in a perfume compound. Examples include Quelques Fleurs by Houbigant and Joy by Jean Patou.
- Ambered, or "Oriental": A large fragrance class featuring the sweet slightly animalic scents of amber-

gris or labdanum, often combined with vanilla, tonka bean, flowers and woods. Can be enhanced by camphorous oils and incense resins, which bring to mind Victorian era imagery of the Middle East and Far East. Traditional examples include Guerlain's Shalimar and Yves Saint Laurent's Opium.

- Wood: Fragrances that are dominated by woody scents, typically of agarwood, sandalwood and cedarwood. Patchouli, with its camphoraceous smell, is commonly found in these perfumes. A traditional example here would be Myrurgia's Maderas De Oriente or Chanel Bois-des-Îles. A modern example would be Balenciaga Rumba.

- Leather: A family of fragrances which features the scents of honey, tobacco, wood and wood tars in its middle or base notes and a scent that alludes to leather. Traditional examples include Robert Piguet's Bandit and Balmain's Jolie Madame.

- Chypre: Meaning Cyprus in French, this includes fragrances built on a similar accord consisting of bergamot, oakmoss, patchouli, and labdanum. This family of fragrances is named after a perfume by François Coty, and one of the most famous examples is Guerlain's Mitsouko.

- Fougère: Meaning Fern in French, built on a base of lavender, coumarin and oakmoss. Houbigant's Fougère Royale pioneered the use of this base. Many men's fragrances belong to this family of fragrances, which is characterized by its sharp herbaceous and woody scent. Some well-known modern fougères are Fabergé Brut and Guy Laroche Drakkar Noir. [5]

The Years 1900–1920

In 1900, the "art nouveau" was embraced with enthusiasm. Thriving fragrance industries turned out luxurious products with prestigious names in artistic bottles.

Coty, a gifted visionary, teamed up with the equally talented Lalique and created a truly luxurious product: La Belle Epoque. They captured the romance of this bygone era in a spicy illusion of clove-scented carnation petals.

Beauty care and cosmetic pioneers, Elizabeth Arden and Helena Rubinstein, opened their fashion doors and later added fragrance to fulfill their customers' requests.

The Years 1920–1930

During the extravagant years of the Roaring Twenties, flappers embraced emancipation and innovation with gusto! The novel freshness of aldehydic fragrances was discovered.

There was a feeling of giddy lightness, and the stars of silent movies made everyone swoon. Chanel No. 5 and Guerlain's Shalimar were both launched and remain as classic favorites in today's market.

The Years 1930–1950

> After World War II, Haute Couture and fragrance combined to create an image of feminine seduction inspired by Hollywood.[6]

Visible signs of change were found in Christian Dior's weekly magazine, *Marie Claire*. Widely distributed, it had sections dedicated to fashion and beauty. Designers created "character fragrances," and one wore designer fragrances to stand out.

The design house of Jean Patou launched Joy Perfume, classified as a refined, flowery fragrance recommended for evening. It includes rare oils of jasmine and rose.

Italian brands created fragrances for Cary Crant, David Niven, Ava Gardner, and Audrey Hepburn. Acqua Di Parma Profumo, a woman's chypre fragrance, is a truly elegant and sophisticated perfume. It was relaunched in 2000 and is considered as chic as "a little black dress with pearls."

Modern Scents Emerge

Since 1945, new categories have emerged to describe modern scents due to great advances in the technology of perfume creation as well as the natural development of styles and tastes.

- Bright Floral: combining the traditional Single Floral and Floral Bouquet categories. A good example would be Estée Lauder's Beautiful.
- Green: a lighter and more modern interpretation of the Chypre type, with pronounced cut grass, crushed green leaf and cucumber-like scents. Two examples would be Estée Lauder's Aliage or Sisley's Eau de Campagne.
- Aquatic, Oceanic, or Ozonic: the newest category in perfume history, appearing in 1991 with Christian Dior's Dune. A very clean, modern smell leading to many of the modern androgynous perfumes. Generally contains calone, a synthetic scent discovered in 1966. Also used to accent floral, oriental, and woody fragrances.
- Citrus: an old fragrance family that until recently consisted mainly of "freshening" eau de colognes, due to the low tenacity of citrus scents. Develop-

ment of newer fragrance compounds has allowed for the creation of primarily citrus fragrances. A good example here would be Brut.

- Fruity: featuring the aromas of fruits other than citrus, such as peach, cassis (black currant), mango, passion fruit, and others. A modern example here would be Ginestet Botrytis.
- Gourmand (French): scents with "edible" or "dessert"-like qualities. These often contain notes like vanilla, tonka bean and coumarin, as well as synthetic components designed to resemble food flavors. A sweet example is Thierry Mugler's Angel. A savory example would be Dinner by BoBo, which has cumin and curry hints. [7]

The Years 1950–1960

During the fifties, fragrance lost its exclusive image, and Europe looked longingly toward America's modern influence and relaxed lifestyle. Fragrances too were becoming more accessible and began to appeal to a wider audience.

The first eau de toilette for men emerged with discreetly elegant notes of lavender and vetiver. Estée Lauder launched the first American fragrance for women, named Estée after herself.

The Years 1960–1970

1960 ushered in an era of opposition and a change in social behavior. In terms of fragrance, it signaled the appearance of a new olfactive freshness.[8]

The hippy movement of the sixties sprang up in San Francisco and sparked a sexual revolution. There was a growing awareness of the body and its five senses along with a rebellious mood of "make love, not war." Patchouli once again invaded the streets.

The Years 1970–1980

> The seventies woman claimed her individuality and proudly wore a lifestyle scent. Men started to use scent independently of their grooming/shaving ritual.[9]

The most important factor in fragrance was the lifestyle message it reflected of feminism, back to nature, gay, punk, and neoromanticism.

New provocative and sophisticated fragrances as well as soft romantic scents wooed women. Men no longer viewed fragrance as simply "aftershave," and true men's cologne began to appear on the market.

The Years 1980–1990

This was a time of unabashed individualism and confrontational personalities. It was reflected with strong fragrances that symbolized personal power.

> Men's fragrances exalted the male body as it confronted the natural elements. Women, on the other hand, wore power suits and overly strong fragrances to broadcast their professional success. New fruity notes, which originated in the US, added a novel twist to men's and women's fragrances.[10]

The Years 1990–2000

Men and women began to yearn for a purer world, and materialism faded as people began to embrace the New

Age lifestyle. The Internet expanded to create the birth of an interplanetary village that touched every aspect of our lives.

Some perfumes linked taste and smell to sweet youthful memories of vanilla, cream, and caramel that soothed societal fears that ended the Millennium. Other fragrances evoked the basic scents of earth, wind, fire, and water. This satisfied the desire for a new natural freshness for both men and women.

The Years 2000–2008

> After the 90s' search for simplicity, sheerness and purity, the 21st century has focused on a return of the entrepreneur and the desire to control your own destiny.[11]

Torrid world events created a shock wave that brought about a search for instant gratification. Social networking on the Internet has created a global village that connects ecocitizens.

The success of gourmand orientals, initiated by Angel, marches on, but the fragrance world begins to lean toward a vintage concept expressed in nouveaux chypres, like Coco Mademoiselle, modernized with fruity florals.

Men's fragrances explore an intense spicy woods, and even floral sensuality. Unisex fragrances go on the market as well as limited-edition, exclusive, and vintage fragrances to satisfy a desire to stand out from the crowd.

And to satisfy this desire, fragrance is going all out with limited-edition, exclusive, vintage (in the sense of specifying the year of creation, like fine wines), and even custom-made scents.

According to Catherine Capozzi, an eHow contributor,

> The perfume industry earns billions yearly! A 2009 New York Times article estimates the perfume industry rakes in annual sales at an astounding $25 to $30 billion. The article states that 83 percent of women wear perfume occasionally and 36 percent wear fragrance every day. This powerhouse industry owes its success to extensive marketing, high profit margins and careful customer targeting.[12]

Vintage Ads

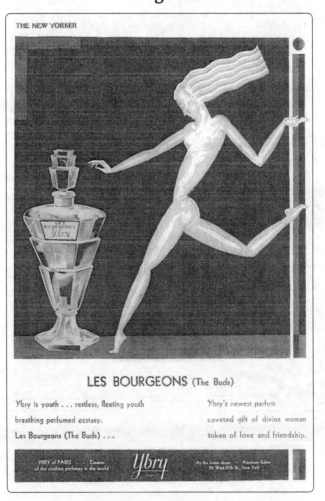

1920s, Les Bourgeons, Ybry

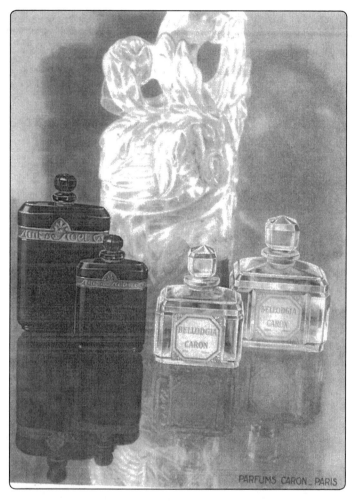

1920s, Bellodgia, Parfums Caron

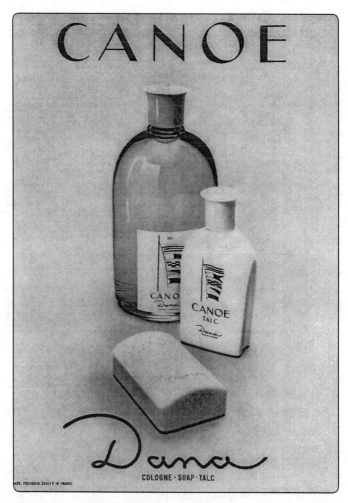

1930s, Canoe, Dana

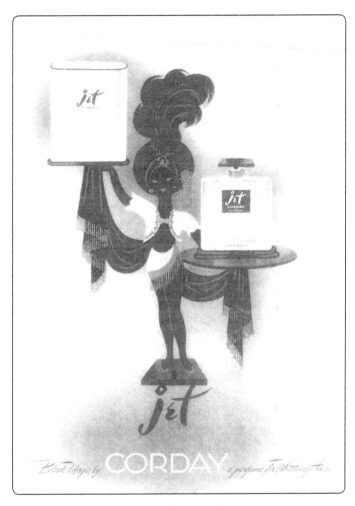

1940s, Jet, Corday

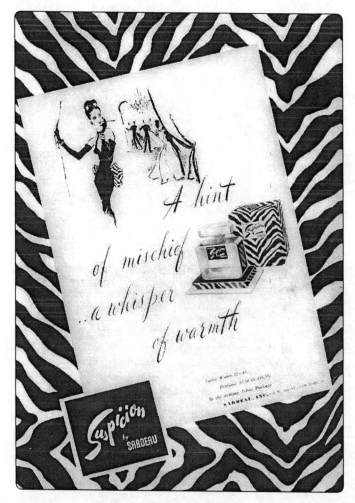

1940s, Suspicion, Sardeau

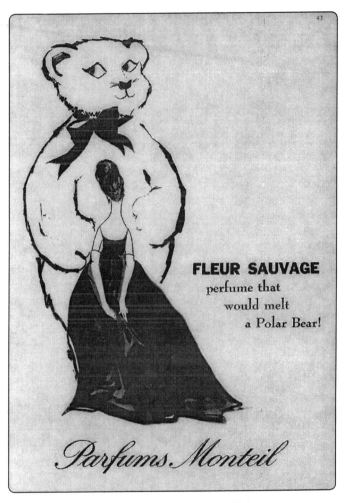

1950s, Fleur Savage, Parfums Monteil

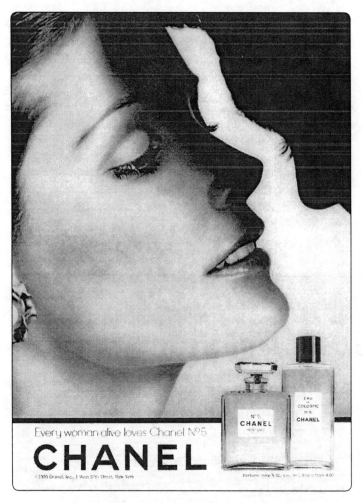

1970s, Chanel No 5, Chanel

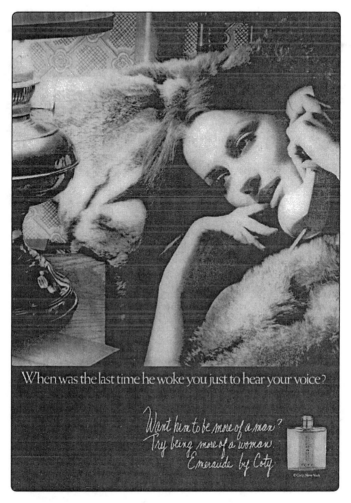

1970s, Emeraude, Coty

I found these old advertisements on a vintage poster sites that also includes other art posters from movies, sports, animals, celebrities, famous people, and more.[13]

2

The Buzz about Blood Types

It interests me to notice how much blood types have become increasingly popular in current discussions. Although there is no proven correlation between blood type and personality, it is a popular belief. Some of today's magazines feature the Japanese belief that a person's ABO blood type is predictive of their personality, temperament, and compatibility with others. Some morning television shows and daily newspapers actually feature blood type horoscopes.

Today in our Western world, many companies and corporations, both large and small, use a standard personality test as part of their hiring process. Potential employees are categorized as types A, B, C, and D. When you compare them to blood types, you can also see a definite correlation between the two.

However, after years of experience in the fragrance world, I have come to the conclusion that there is definitely something to how much our blood types determine our actions and reactions. I am also convinced that we are born with certain personality traits that are determined by our blood type.

This chapter deals with the discovery of blood types and gives readers a look at international blood types and the initial study by the Japanese about their observation of temperaments through blood type.

The Discovery of Blood Types

Did you know that the four main blood types were not discovered until the early 1900s? O was determined to be the original type and is the largest universal blood type in over 40 percent of the world's population. As people began to farm and explore the world, the A and B types developed. The AB blood type is the newest and is only about five hundred years old!

As research continued, important differences were discovered concerning the blood types.

> Biologists could not understand why some transfusions worked and others didn't. Sometimes the patients lived, and sometimes they had bad reactions. In 1909, Karl Landsteiner in Vienna, Austria made the discovery that all blood is not alike. He won the Nobel Peace Prize for his work. There were four main groupings of blood—A, B, AB, and O—and they were not all compatible with each other. Since then, over 300 blood types have been discovered, all falling into one of these four major groups.[1]

The relevance of this to perfume is that your blood carries the micronutrients that create your personal body chemistry. "These nutrients perform various functions, including the building of bones and cell structures, regulating the body's pH, carrying charge, and driving chemical reactions."[2]

A Few Worldwide Blood Types

Next, I've listed a few blood type percentages that indicate nationality and probable blood type. Taken from Wikipedia, these numbers are disputed due to more recent studies; however, this is just a partial worldwide list of ABO numbers to consider and compare.[3]

- Australia: O–41%, A–38%, B–10%, AB–3%
- Canada: O–46%, A–42 %, B–9%, AB–3%
- France, Germany, Spain (avg): O–42%, A–44%, B–10%, AB–4%
- Hong Kong: O–40%, A–26%, B–27%, AB–7%
- India: O–38%, A–23%, B–32%, AB–7%
- Japan: O–31%, A–40%, B–20%, AB–9%
- S. Africa: O–46%, A–37%, B–14%, AB–4%
- United Kingdom and United States (avg): O–44%, A–42%, B–10%, AB–4%

Blood Type Personalities

While researching my theory, I came across this popular system that categorizes people according to blood types. It dates back to 1927 when it was first proposed by a Japanese psychology professor, Furukawa Takeji.

Furukawa was a high school administrator who began to observe the differences in temperament of the school's students. He published a paper called "The Study of Temperament through Blood Type" in the journal *Psychological Research*. Despite a lack of hard evidence, the public gobbled up ketsueki-gata (blood type), but after Furukawa's death in 1940, the interest waned.

Ketsueki-gata was revived again in 1971 when a journalist, Masahiko Nomi, expanded on Furukawa's theories. Nomi's new theories associated some blood types to academic success and even different types of crimes.

After Mashiko Nomi's death, his son, Toshitaka, continued these studies and founded the Institute of Blood Type Humanics, and interest in ketsueki-gata has continued to grow.[4]

British writer Ruth Evans reported, "Its purpose is not to stereotype people but to study how to make the best of their talents and improve human relationships. Together, father and son have written dozens of books on the subject."[5]

I am fascinated by all of this and tend to agree that there is definitely something to it. Anyway, it's interesting reading.

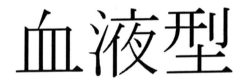

Descriptions of Blood Type Personalities

As I continued my search, I came across several articles about blood type personalities. I found this example on the blog site The Great Greek Manual. I think these descriptions are really close to what I have observed.

Type A: The Farmer

Type A people are calm, composed, levelheaded, and very serious. They have a firm character, and are reliable, trustworthy, and hardheaded. They are shy, introverted perfectionists. They are considerate to others and don't easily lie. They are loyal to friends and coworkers. They can be secretive, though, and don't often share their feelings. They try to suppress their own emotions, and because they have continual practice in doing this, they appear strong, when in actuality, they have a fragile, nervous side, as well. They tend to be hard on people who are not of the same type, and consequently, tend to be surrounded with people of the same temperament. They also don't hold their liquor well.

Type A's are the most artistic of the groups. They can be shy, cautious, conscientious, reliable, trustworthy, and sensitive. They can also be overcautious, picky, arrogant, and reckless when drunk.

Type B: The Hunter

People with Type B Blood are curious everything. That may be good, but they also tend to have too many interests and hobbies. They tend to get excited about something suddenly only to drop it again just as quickly. They seem to manage to know which of their many interests or loved ones are truly the most important. B Types tend to excel in things rather than just be average, but they tend to be so involved in their own world that they neglect other things. They have independent spirits with strong personalities. They have the image of being bright and cheerful, full of energy and enthusiasm, but some people think that they are really quite different on the inside. They also don't really want to have much personal contact with others. While they don't care what others think of them. They are extremely passionate about the things they hold dear.

Type B's are the individualists of the blood group categories and find their own way in life. Type B personalities can be curious, bright, cheerful, enthusiastic, independent, sensitive, and unpredictable. They can also be superficial, unreliable, selfish, unpredictable, indiscreet, lazy and impatient

Type AB: The Humanist

Type AB people are an unpredictable, distant lot, but tend to use their heads over their hearts. They are good with money. They are considerate of other people's feelings and deal with them with care and caution. On the other hand, though, they are strict with themselves and those close to them. They, therefore, seem to have two personalities: one for those "outside," and another for people on the "inside." They often become sentimental, and they tend to think too deeply about things. AB Types have a lot of friends, but they need time to be alone and think things through, as well. They can be both outgoing and shy, confident and timid. While responsible, too much responsibility will cause a problem. They are trustworthy and like to help others.

Type AB's are the split-personalities of the blood groups. They can be sensitive, considerate, careful, and efficient, however; they can also be strict, moody, easily offended, critical, and standoffish.

Type O: The Warrior

Type O people are outgoing, expressive and passionate. They are highly motivated, natural leaders. Blessed with a strong physical presence, they aren't afraid to gamble because they are so convinced they'll win. Type O Blood people are said to set the mood for a group and to take on the role of creating harmony among its members. Their image is one of being peaceful and carefree. They are also thought to be big-hearted and benevolent, and they tend to spend money on others generously.

They are natural athletes. They tend to be obsessive in their quest for success, and this can make them boring to others. Type O's are outgoing, and very social. They are initiators, although they don't always finish what they start. They appear to be levelheaded and trustworthy, but they often slip and make big blunders inadvertently. That is also the what makes O Types lovable. Creative and popular, they love to be the center of attention and appear very self-confident.

Type O personalities are the natural leaders. They can be carefree, generous, independent, flexible, idealistic, goal-oriented, athletic, competitive, and adaptable. They can also be clumsy, flighty, jealous, greedy, unreliable, obsessive lover, vain loudmouths.[6]

Modern Personality Types

Today in our Western world, many companies and corporations use a standard personality test as part of their hiring process to determine the applicant's type. Interestingly enough, these modern career personality types are classified into four types—A, B, C, and D. These can be correlated to blood types.

When compared, I did see a definite pattern between the two. This information led me to confirm my belief in the parallels between personality and blood types, commonly called "body chemistry."

The first about blood types is by Natalie Josef. I really liked how she expresses her findings about ABO types and personalities. I have indicated beside the blood types what I also think are their matching personality types.

I totally agree with this ABO fan's comment: "Relation between blood type and personality, results differ by questionnaires."

But we both agree that there is a consistent relation, although it's not yet definitely proven due to random sampling methods. A closer look at social position, age, and regions will be necessary to get more accurate and stable results. Let's hope that for the average consumer, these studies will become serious research that will enlighten us to the facts about these parallels and then how they match up in the fragrance world. Until then, my opinions are based upon personal observations, experience, and the curiosity about genetic markers found in our blood.

Most people have at least heard of this basic personality concept of being either hard-driving or laid-back and seem to lean to one side or the other with regards to the Type A (dominant) or B (passive) division.

The Spin on Personality

Blood Type O
Basic Personality A = Modern Type A

You are the social butterflies. Often popular and self-confident, you are very creative and always seem to be the center of attention. You make a good impression on people and you're often quite attractive. Organized and determined, your stubbornness will help you reach your goals. You make good leaders.

Common career choices: banker, politician, gambler, minister, investment broker, and pro athlete

Lovewise, O is most compatible with O and AB.

Blood Type A
Basic Personality B = Modern Type C

Type A's may seem calm on the outside, but inside, you're filled with anxiety and worry. You're perfectionists and often shy and sensitive. Usually introverted, you're stable and thoughtful. You make good listeners and are sensitive to color and your surroundings. You like to be fashionable and are up on the latest trends, but never flashy or gaudy. You like romantic settings and often shun reality for fantasy worlds.

Common career choices: accountant, librarian, economist, writer, computer programmer, and gossip columnist

Lovewise, A is most compatible with A and AB in the love department.

Blood Type B
Basic Personality A = Modern Type B

You can be very goal-oriented and often complete the ambitious tasks set before you. Outgoing and very charming, you're good at reading people and providing support. Though critical of appearance (but not your own), you aren't picky and are unlikely to dwell over the little things. Type B's are impulsive.

Common career choices: cook, hairdresser, military leader, talk show host, and journalist

Lovewise, B is most compatible with B and AB lovers.

Blood Type AB
Basic Personality B = Modern Type D

Not surprisingly, AB's can be quite dualistic, possessing both A and B traits. You may be shy and outgoing, and hesitant and confident. You often stand out from others, don't like labels, and are nice and easy going. You are logical and determined to do things correctly. Usually trustworthy, you like to help others. You often speak in a serious manner. Your patience, concentration, and intelligence are admirable.

Common career choices: bartender, lawyer, teacher, sales representative, and social worker

Lovewise: AB can find a soul mate with any other blood type.[7]

This is how my theory spins. To unravel this mystery, you can compare the ABO blood types with personality types. Identifiable personality types have been developed by advances in the field of psychology to understand human behavior. Four major types have been categorized that group individuals based on their behavior.

My theory matches the four blood types and behavioral groups that are subsequently mirrored in fragrance choices. I found the following online at Buzzle.com. I've noted ABO blood type beside the personality type.

Personality Type A
"Bulldozers" (Blood Type O)

The individuals that come under personality type A are of a highly independent nature. These can best be described as the Bulldozers. Their ambition to leave their mark in this world singles them out. They are self-driven and know the importance of goal setting, positive thinking and motivation.

If you are interested in studying a specimen of this type, choose one from the ranks of business leadership. They are competitive in nature, in fact they thrive on it as if it is the fuel of their life. They are well-known for their sharpness in getting to the heart of the matter in no-nonsense and blunt terms. Individuals of personality type A are risk takers which characterizes an entrepreneurial spirit. They do have the ability to put on the veil of practicality to solve a problem as and when it is required. The secret of these successful people is that they don't balk under the requirements and necessity of change which eventually, make them what they want to be.

Personality Type B
"Bombers" (Blood Type B)

These people can be described as the Bombers. These characters are extroverts to the soles of their boots, and think, that life is nothing else but getting under the spotlight and spell binding the rest. Individuals that fall under this category are human magnets that can attract attention of everyone in a gathering without so much of an effort. This makes them special, among the various other personalities.

These people have a very engaging personality, and when it comes to conversations they are as sleek as eels and as voluminous as the Niagara Falls.

Individuals can sell a fridge to an Eskimo who, after the sale, thanks all his departed ancestors and the snowman for bestowing the honor of buying something from this wonderful man. Because of their ability to get tuned in with the people, others find them a fountain of entertainment and charisma. Turn and focus your microscope to sales and marketing fields or to those people in the field of entertainment and you will find them in no time. They thrive on the interactions with the others. Your act of ignoring them or their efforts is as good as you sticking a knife in their back, for them. Not being able to attract your attention or making you sway to their tune, hurts these people.

Personality Type C
"Seekers" (Blood Type A)

The apt term to describe these people is the Seekers. If you are searching for a promising heir to your microscope to bestow on, you can choose any person of personality type C. These are the introverts interested in details which separates them from the rest of the types. They could turn heaven and hell upside down or inside-out, depending on their mood, to find a fact they are interested in, before taking it to pieces in order to restart the process.

These people tend to shrink from social or human interaction. Arranging facts (which include women and their behavior) around them, in a logical order is what drives these people to no end. A person of this type can live with an individual of personality type B, as happily as a meditative ton of matter with an outgoing, bubbling, jesting and noisy ton of antimatter. Big Bang? Yes, type C is as exactly opposite of type B as an electron with the left spin is the antithesis of the one with the right spin.

You can find specimens of type C personified in accountants, computer programmers, etc. These people find it difficult to get out of their shell and communicate with other people, but are tigers when it comes to numbers and logic. Reserved nature is the mark of type C, and they are cautious, too. Risk taking is not a very attractive option for these people who tend not to venture into something until, they have gone over all the facts with a fine toothed comb.

Personality Type D
"Followers" (Blood Type AB)

These gentlemen really believe in inertia which they have no shortage of. These people prefer to stick to the trodden paths and established routines over the uncertainty of change. You will find, ... a true specimen of this type in people engaged as clerks.

These are Followers of the spent actions and executors of the direct commands. You will find them doing their best not to stretch their neck out when it comes to taking responsibility and risk. With the help of professionals in the field of personality development and through sheer power of self motivation or self-improvement, these people can overcome their handicap to some extent.

These individuals are afflicted by negativity such as worry, irritability, gloom, etc., and hardly feel self-assured. To avoid rejection, they avoid to open up and share their negative emotions. This causes them to suffer from enormous amount of stress which makes them prone to heart related diseases. The studies show that as many as 18 to 53 percent of cardiac patients have type D personality.[7]

The following is one of my favorite findings by Natalie Josef, a writer who blogged about blood types determining your personalities back in 2008.[9]

I really liked how she expressed her findings about ABO types and personalities. I have indicated beside the blood types matching personality types, common career choices, their most compatible love match and best and worst traits.

Blood Type O: Warrior
Basic Personality A = Modern Type A

Career: banker, politician, gambler, minister, investment broker, and pro athlete

Lovewise: O is most compatible with O and AB.

Best Traits: Agreeable, sociable, optimistic
Worst Traits: Vain, rude, jealous

Blood Type A: Farmer
Basic Personality B = Modern Type C

Career: accountant, librarian, economist, writer, computer programmer

Lovewise: A is most compatible with A and AB in the love department.

Best Traits: Creative, patient, reserved, responsible
Worst Traits: Fastidious, stubborn, tense

Blood Type B: Hunter
Basic Personality A = Modern Type B

Career: cook, hairdresser, military leader,
talk show host, and journalist

Lovewise: B is most compatible with B and AB lovers.

Best Traits: Strong, creative, passionate
Worst Traits: Selfish, unforgiving, unpredictable

Blood Type AB: Humanist
Basic Personality B = Personality Type D

Career: bartender, lawyer, teacher, sales
representative, and social worker

Lovewise: AB can find a soul mate
with any other blood type.

Best Traits: Cool, sociable, adaptable
Worst Traits: Critical, indecisive, forgetful

Thinking More about My Theory

So we've gained awareness of blood type personalities.

My thinking is that with four basic blood and personality types, there has to be a correlation to the fragrance families. All three of these branch out, but their commonality is that there are basically four of each. And I've decided that all three are parallel!

To challenge my theory, I decided to create my own "scent-sational survey." I collected over two hundred of them, and it comes out to be between 80 to 90 percent accurate. And folks, that is strong when you figure a 6 to 8 percent margin of error! I've included a survey copy in this chapter.

The survey asks about blood type, fave fragrances, and personalities. Its main purpose was to help determine a fragrance family match that could help direct people to better perfume choices.

The trick is to identify the blood type and/or personality. Then refer to my new fragrance chart to help determine the best fragrance family for an individual.

I found this short survey to be very helpful since some people have no clue about their blood type. Some cannot decide about their personality type. I made this into my game, and it's a great place to start your fragrance search. Try it now.

Scent-sational Survey

1. What is your blood type?
   O _____ A _____ B _____ AB _____

2. What types of fragrances do you prefer? (Please number 1, 2, 3, 4 in order of preference.)
   _____ (Typical O) floral, woodsy, spicy
   _____ (Typical A) fruity floral
   _____ (Typical B) crisp citrus, fresh outdoor scent
   _____ (Typical AB) delicate floral/powdery

3. List your favorite top three fragrances.
   _____
   _____
   _____

4. Check which one best describes your personality?
____ Type O: natural leaders. Can be carefree, generous, independent, flexible, idealistic, goal-oriented, athletic, competitive, and adaptable
____ Type A: the most artistic of the groups. Can be shy, cautious, conscientious, reliable, trustworthy, and sensitive
____ Type B: these individualists can be curious, bright, cheerful, enthusiastic, independent, sensitive, and unpredictable.
____ Type AB: the split personalities of the blood groups. Can be sensitive, considerate, careful and efficient. On the other hand, they can also be strict, moody, easily offended, critical, and standoffish.

After you have taken the survey, refer to my fragrance chart in chapter 6 and the cross-references listed in chapter 9 for fragrances that should be good choices. Keep in mind that this is not a proven theory and that body chemistries can differ for many reasons, such as age, hormones, and diet.

Also, when thinking about the notes in fragrances, keep in mind that the amounts vary in different compositions. For example, I have observed that one may not be a big fan of vanilla but that just a small amount will create a softness that O and AB blood types seem to like. Too much vanilla seems to turn them away.

3

Four Basic Fragrance Families

Even with all the information and scientific determinations of fragrance categories, I find they can still be separated into four basic families. To simplify the matter of finding a fragrance family for an individual, I chose to work from this point of view as a basic starting place.

The more I read and studied, the more I realized that having an understanding about fragrance classifications is good information to know.

What you initially smell when testing a perfume is not necessarily what you might expect as an end result. I believe this is due to how the body reacts to the notes. So learning what scents do or do not work for a person can be very helpful.

I strongly agree with the following information from The Perfumed Court website, which is a great place to buy perfume samples. They referenced this information to Osmoz.

According to Osmoz, there are eight major families: chypre, citrus, floral, and oriental (feminine), and aromatic, citrus, oriental, and woody (masculine). Each one of those olfactive families is then split into several subfamilies.[1]

Women's Counter

1. CHYPRE—Based on a woody, mossy, floral accord, which can include leathery or fruity notes as well. Chypre perfumes have a rich and lingering scent. Chypre by Coty enjoyed such success in 1917 that "chypre" is now a generic name for a whole category of classic perfumes. The compositions are based on oakmoss, ciste-labdanun, patchouli and bergamot accords. The richness of chypre notes mixes wonderfully with fruity or floral notes. This family is made up of distinguished, instantly recognizable fragrances.

   Subgroups under this family are Floral and Fruity:

   • Floral—floral notes such as lily of the valley, rose or jasmine are added to the chypre structure. Examples include: Badgley Mischka, Clinique Aromatics Elixir, Givenchy Amariage Mariage, Chanel Chance and Donna Karan DKNY Be Delicious
   • Fruity—The chypre accord is enriched and embellished with fruity notes such as peach, mirabelle plum and exotic fruit. Examples include: Chanel Coco Mademoiselle, Guerlain Mitsouko, and Dior Miss Dior Cherie.

2. Citrus—Each perfume in this family is primarily composed of citrus scents such as bergamot, lemon, orange, tangerine and grapefruit, to which other orange-tree elements (orange blossoms, petit grain or neroli oil) have been added. Floral or even chypre accords are sometimes present as well. These perfumes are characterized by their freshness and lightness including the first "Eaux de Cologne."

   The one subgroup under this family is Aromatic.

   • Aromatic—The citrus accord is enhanced by the addition of aromatic notes, such as thyme, rosemary, tarragon or mint. Examples include: Calvin Klein CK One, Rochas Eau de Rochas, and Lancome O de Lancome.

3. Floral—This family is composed of a large variety of creations ranging from sumptuous bouquet arrangements to 'soli flora' compositions. Perfumers can let their creativity run wild, enriching florals with green, aldehydic, fruity or spicy hints. With its natural scent, the floral note is one of the most widely used in women's perfumes.

   Subgroups under this family are Aldehyde, Aquatic, Carnation, Fruity, Green, Jasmine, Muguet, Orange Tuberose, Rose Violet and Woody Musk:

   • Aldehyde—Animal, powdery or slightly woody notes often enhance the floral bouquet. The top note is a marriage of aldehydes and hesperidia. This sub-family came into existence with the creation of Chanel No. 5, the first floral-aldehydic perfume with an unusually high amount of aldehydes. Examples include: Chanel No. 5 and Estée Lauder White Linen.

- Aquatic—A traditional floral bouquet is enhanced with several marine notes during the evaporation process. Examples include: Aramis New West for Her, Davidoff Cool Water Woman, Issey Miyake L'Eau d'Issey for Women, Davidoff Cool Water Game Woman, and Escada Into the Blue.
- Carnation—"The poet's flower" is also found in perfumery and plays a part in the development of rich and harmonious fragrances. Examples include: Calvin Klein Eternity for Women, Nina Ricci L'Air du Temps and Lancome Miracle.
- Green—Green notes can add a sharper freshness to the floral bouquet. Galbanum is a typical ingredient in this type of perfume as well as combinations that evoke freshly-cut grass. Examples include: Chanel No. 19, Ralph Lauren Lauren, and Estée Lauder Beautiful.
- Fruity—Since 1995, new fruity notes have blossomed in the world of perfumery. The floral body is easily identifiable, and the fruity notes are obvious. Among these are apricot, raspberry, lychee and apple. Examples include: Armani Acqua di Gio, Cacharel Amor Amor, Carolina Herrera 212, Clinique Happy, Armani Emporio Remix for Her, Cacharel Noa Perle, Cartier Delices, Dior J'Adore, Escada Pacific Paradise, Juicy Couture, Vera Wang Princess, Guerlain Insolence, and Nina Ricci Nina.

- Jasmine—Also know as "The Flower," jasmine enhances the floral top notes. It helps give perfume a complex and refined structure. Examples include: Burberry London, Ferragamo F, Dior Pure Poison and Jean Patou Joy.
- Muguet—A floral bouquet whose keynote is lily of the valley, a timeless white flower which gives perfume a fresh note of springtime. Examples include: Cacharel Anais Anais and Estée Lauder Pleasures for Women.
- Orange Tuberose—Introduced in 1948 with Fracas de Piguet, this sub-family has kept all of its appeal. It includes original scents of a unique sensuality. Examples include: Armani Code for Her and Givenchy Amarige.
- Rose Violet—The key floral accord of this sub-family is rose and violet. This widely used flower duet was launched by Paris, the famous Yves Saint Laurent perfume. Examples include: Lancome Tresor and Yves Saint Laurent Paris.
- Woody Musk—Always based on a floral accord, this family includes fragrances with an additional woody and/or musky note, which gives a richer, more contemporary structure than that of a traditional floral perfume. Examples include: Aramis Always for Her, Calvin Klein CK, Lanvin Rumeur, Bulgari Blv, Donna Karan Gold, Kenzo Kenzo Amour, Lucky Brand Number 6 for Women, Sarah Jessica Parker Lovely and Stella McCartney Stella in Two Peony.

4. Oriental—Also known as "amber" fragrances—stand out because of their unique blend of warmth

and sensuality. They draw their richness from heady substances like musk, vanilla and precious woods, often associated with exotic floral and spicy scents. Subgroups under this family are: Floral, Spicy, Vanilla and Woody.

- Floral—Traditional Oriental base composed of sweet, powdery element, accompanies by an exotic floral note such as tiare flower or "spicy" flowers such as carnation. Examples include: Britney Spears In Control Curious, Dolce and Gabbana The One, Gaultier Jean-Paul Gaultier, Guerlain L'Heure Bleu, Calvin Klein Euphoria, Donna Karan Cashmere Mist, Givenchy Ange ou Demon, Guerlain L'Instant de Guerlain, Tom Ford Black Orchid, Van Cleef and Arpels First Love, Kenzo Flower by Kenzo, and Stella McCartney Stella In Two Amber.
- Spicy—Spices such as cinnamon, cloves and nutmeg join the Oriental accord to enhance the originality and character of these unmistakable perfumes. Examples include: Chanel Coco, Sonia Rykiel Belle en Rykiel, Estée Lauder Youth Dew and Yves Saint Laurent Opium.
- Vanilla—Vanilla and classical amber notes accentuate the original Oriental aroma. Examples include: Armani Emporio She, Chanel Allure, Guerlain Shalimar, Lolita Lempicka "L," Ralph Lauren Ralph Hot, Calvin Klein Obsession, Dior Hypnotic Poison, Lancome Miracle Forever, and Thierry Mugler Angel.

- Woody—Warm and opulent notes like amber and sandalwood, or dry notes like cedar are added to the Oriental accord to further accentuate it. Examples include: Bulgari Eau Parfume au The Rouge, Lancome Hypnose, Thierry Mugler Alien, Guerlain Samsar and Molinard Habanita.

Men's Counter

1. Aromatic—Aromatic notes are mainly composed of sage, rosemary, thyme and lavender usually complemented with citrus and spicy notes. These compositions' manly character makes them an all-time favorite in men's perfumery.

   Subgroups under this family are Aquatic, Fougere, Fresh and Rustic.

   - Aquatic—The compositions of this subfamily brighten up the basic aromatic accord with an ocean note. This modern family boasts many recent creations. Examples include: Armani Acqua Di Gio for Men, Davidoff Cool Water Game, Bulgari AQVA Pour Homme and Kenzo for Men.

   - Fougere—Timeless aromatic notes blend with a traditional fougere accord characterized by lavender, woody, coumarin, geranium and oak moss notes. Examples include: Armani Emporio Remix for Him, Dolce and Gabbana Classique, Guy Laroche Drakkar Noir, Loewe Escenia Loewe, Azzaro Pour Homme, Faberge Brut Original, Hugo Boss BOSS Selection, and Lucky Brand 6 for Men.

- Fresh—Fresh notes such as white flowers or citrus notes are added to an aromatic bouquet characterized by an underlying woody note. Examples include: Calvin Klein Eternity for Men, Davidoff Cool Water, Liz Claiborne Curve for Men, Clinique Happy for Men, Estée Lauder Pleasures for Men, Tommy Hilfiger T.
- Rustic—The dominant aromatic accord is enhanced by the addition of rustic notes carrying scents of the countryside such as new-mown hay or grass. Examples include: Aramis New West for Men, Hugo Boss Hugo, Ralph Lauren Polo Sport, Calvin Klein Escape for Men and Kenneth Cole Reaction.

2. Citrus—This family includes all perfumes mainly composed of citrus notes such as bergamot, lemon, orange, tangerine and grapefruit. These fragrances are characterized by their freshness and lightness. The first Eaux de Cologne belong to this category. The masculine character comes from the frequently strong presence of aromatic and spicy notes.
   The one subgroup under this family is Aromatic.

- Aromatic—The hesperidium accord is enhanced by the addition of aromatic notes, such as thyme, rosemary or tarragon. Examples include: Armani Pour Homme, Dior Eau Sauvage and Azzaro Chrome.

3. Oriental—Refreshed by aromatic or citrus facets, Oriental compositions draw their richness and sophistication from precious substances such as

amber, resin, tobacco, spices, exotic woods and animal notes.

Subgroups under this family are Fougere, Spicy and Woody.

- Fougere—These timeless Oriental fragrances emanate a traditional top note of fern scent composed of lavender, coumarin, and oak moss. Examples include: Gaultier Le Male, Joop Homme, Hugo Boss Boss in Motion and Prada Pour Homme.
- Spicy—A distinct spicy note livens up the amber accord with nutmeg, cloves, cinnamon or cardamom. Examples include: Armani Code, Cartier Must for Men, Hugo Boss Hugo Dark Blue, Burberry London for Men, Hugo Boss Boss Soul and Yves Saint Laurent Body Kouros.
- Woody—Oriental accords composed of warm and rich notes such as vanilla, coumarin and labdanum ciste are emphasized by opulent woody notes like patchouli, sandalwood or vetiver Examples include: Balenciaga Cristobal for Men, Calvin Klein Contradiction for Men, Cerruti 1991 Black, Davidoff Silver Shadow, Burberry Brit for Men, Calvin Klein Obsession for Men, Chanel Allure Homme, Guerlain Habit Rouge, Thierry Mugler A*Men and Viktor and Rolf Antidote.

4. Woody—These perfumes with their woody middle note, are warm and opulent when based on sandalwood or patchouli. Cedar and vetiver make them dryer. These warn, dry and elegant

masculine accords often contain a dash of citrus or aromatic notes.

Subgroups under this family are Aquatic, Aromatic, Chypre, Floral Musk and Spicy.

- Aquatic—This composition if often harmonized with an aromatic woody accord, and ocean notes complement its structure. Examples include: Aramis Always for Him, Issey Miyake L'Eau d'Issey for Men, Donna Karan Red Delicious Men.
- Aromatic—The woody accords form the core of these compositions and always start on an aromatic note such as thyme, rosemary or sage. Examples include: Azzaro Pure Vetiver, Cerruti 1881 Pour Homme, Kenneth Cole Black for Him, Lacoste Pour Homme, Calvin Klein Euphoria Men, Guerlain Vetiver, Lalique Encre Noire, Yves Saint Laurent Jazz and Ralph Lauren Safari for Men.
- Chypre—The addition of chypre notes such as oakmoss and labdanum ciste enhances the predominant woody accord. Examples include: Aramis and Ralph Lauren Polo.
- Floral Musk—This category is characterized by its predominant woody note, which can either be cedar, patchouli or sandalwood. The diverse floral top notes include violet and freesia. The lingering scent is mostly composed of musky notes. Examples include: Armani Emporio He, Bulgari Pour Homme Soir, Carolina Herrera 212 Men, Burberry Touch for Men, Chanel Egoiste Platinum, Dior Homme, Dior Fahrenheit, Paul Smith for Men, Yves Saint Laurent L'Homme.

- Spicy—A soft sandalwood fragrance warmed by bold spicy notes such as pepper, nutmeg, cloves or cinnamon. Examples include: Armani Mania, Cacharel Amor Pour Homme, Chanel Allure Homme Sport, Gucci Rush for Men, Bulgari Blv Pour Homme, Christian Lacroix Tumulte Pour Homme, Guerlain L'Instant de Guerlain Pour Homme, Hermes Terre d'Hermes, Old Spice Original and Ralph Lauren Polo Double Black.[2]

Scents of Direction

I dare to dream that *Scent-sational Searches* will inspire research that will embrace my theory and produce answers that can, in turn, help the average person find the appropriate fragrance for himself.

When you have discovered the right fragrance family, your sense of smell should conclude that your have found a pleasing, agreeable scent. Also, be aware of your body language when testing a new fragrance. Did you smile and take a second whiff, or did you turn your head away and make a sound that indicated displeasure?

No matter how slight your reaction, your nose knows, and your body *will* talk to you about this matter. *Scent-sational Searches* will help you understand how your body chemistry (blood type) and personality team up to define your search especially when matched up with the fragrance wheel or fragrance chart.

 Buzz Note: Signature scents are specific fragrances by which you may recognize a person. My fave is Chanel No. 5.

4

Get to Know the Fragrance Wheel and Fragranista Chart

During my "scent-sational searches," I came across what is known as the fragrance wheel. It is a relatively new way to classify fragrances, and it is widely used in retail and in the fragrance industry today. I have recently modified this concept into what I have decided to call my fragranista chart. As a bonus, it is inserted into the end of this chapter.

The fragrance wheel itself was a method created in 1983 by Michael Edwards. Edwards is a consultant in the perfume industry who designed his own scheme of fragrance classification after being inspired by a fragrance seminar. The new scheme was created in order to simplify fragrance classification and naming as well as to show the relationships between individual classes. Read more about Edwards in chapter 6, where I have included bios of my fave perfumers.

Fragrance Wheel: Another Factor of Four

After several years of observing customer responses, I had decisive categories of who fit into which fragrance family. After discovering Michael Edward's fragrance wheel, I decided to factor it into my "fragranista theory" as another factor of four to match with the four basic blood types and personality descriptions.

I was just as amazed as the people who played my game as we searched for a perfect fragrance. This all started to make sense! My theory began to come into focus with the fragrance wheel. Searches became easier when we matched blood and/or personality types to one of the four fragrance families.

Edward's original fragrance wheel consisted of five standard families. It included classic categories of floral, oriental, woody, fresh, and fougère.

Fresh consists of newer, bright, and clean-smelling citrus and oceanic fragrances that have arrived due to improvements in fragrance technology. The fougère family was first placed at the center of this wheel since it contains fragrance elements from each of the other four families. During recent revision, it was removed.

The most important thing to notice about the fragrance wheel is that it has four major classifications that break down into fourteen subcategories. In between these are other minor descriptions that indicate more details of the scents.

These are arranged around a wheel to further identify the fragrance families (shown below).

1. Floral: Floral, Soft Floral, Floral Oriental
2. Oriental: Soft Oriental, Oriental, Woody Oriental
3. Woody: Wood, Mossy Woods, Dry Woods
4. Fresh: Citrus, Green, Water[1]

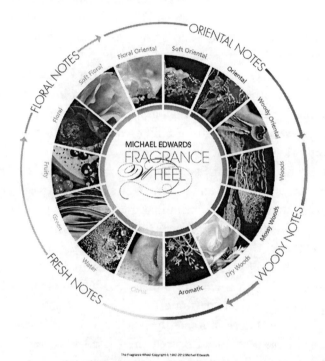

Illustration courtesy of Michael Edwards.

Learn to Use a Fragranista Chart

It is really a quite simple tool that I have created to help you identify fragrance families that relate to blood/personality types. I wish that every fragrance counter had one of these graphics to help simplify choices. Hopefully, one day they will!

Note: For simplicity in the following paragraphs, I am referring only to blood types to match with fragrance families.

People with the O blood type are much, much greater in number and are far more difficult to determine a fragrance preference for than the others. This is also partly due to the fact that there are so many perfumes and other scents to choose from for this group.

O's *do* like heavier, fuller scents. These may include spices and other gourmand notes like spearmint or vanilla. Women's scents vary from light florals (for daytime) to strong woodsy floral (for evening wear). Men float around from oriental to fresh scents.

Even though this family has more difficulty finding fragrances that will remain on their skin and satisfy their senses, their process of elimination becomes much easier when armed with a fragranista chart or fragrance wheel.

I think that perfumers create new fragrances that satisfy these noses first. Whether unknowingly or not, my reasoning is that there are so many more O shoppers who typically love to buy perfume.

In the next exploration of the wheel or chart, A's (women) should look into lines between the top edge of fresh over into the fruity floral. Men would select from fresh bergamot and citrus into aromatic herb toward the woodsy side.

Also under "fresh," the B's, both women and men, will find a small section of crisp green, citrus, and aquatic notes that they enjoy. Only delicate fresh scents will do for the ABs. Women should look for just a whisper of soft floral fragrance or maybe synthetic scents that dry down to powdery notes. The men seem to go for very clean aquatic notes.

These B and AB blood types really struggle to find their perfect scents because there are so few fragrances produced that are good choices for these people. Many would-be fragranistas are super sensitive and do not wear any fragrance because they simply cannot find anything that works for them.

I think that this is mainly due to the fact that they only make up a small fraction of buyers and fewer products are created that they might like. In today's world of marketing, if a product doesn't sell well, it just goes away.

Fragranista Chart: Includes Blood/ Personality Parallels

I have created my own fragranista chart and added my theoretical spin to the wheel by including the blood types, basic personality types (A or B), and modern types (A, B, C, and D) based on American statistics. A copy of my fragranista chart is included below and will be available on the website at DeborahWorley.com

Currently, you can find specific perfumes matched to personality by some companies. However, my fragranista chart indicates the parallels among the blood and personality types to fragrance families. This is intended to bring my theory together for the person in search of the perfect perfume and to help simplify the matter. Take copy of my 'fragranista chart' with you as an aid while you search your fragrance family characteristics.

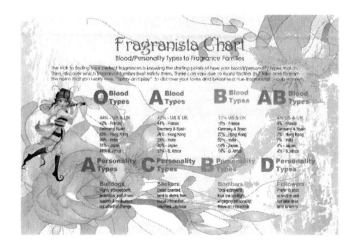

1. Soft Fruity Floral Notes
   (Blood Type A–Basic Personality B/Modern Type C)
   This is a popular category at almost 42 percent. It includes fruit notes and soft floral. However, to me it bridges the water, green, and fruity, which are included in the fresh notes.

2. Fougère, Soft Floral Notes
   (Blood Type AB–Basic Personality B/Modern Type D)
   At 4 percent, this category represents the smallest and newest blood family. This is actually a subcategory that is inside the floral notes family. It does represent an elite group of very sensitive people who do not tolerate heavy or intense smells.

3. Floriental and Woodsy Notes
   (Blood Type O–Basic Personality A/Modern Type A)
   Almost half of the United States population, 44 percent, falls into these two major categories. Minor categories divide into floral oriental, soft

oriental, oriental, woody oriental, woods, mossy woods, and dry woods.

4. Fresh, Aromatic, Citrus Notes
(Blood Type B–Basic Personality A / Modern Type B)
Only 12 percent of the US population fits into this major category. Its minor categories breaks into aromatic, citrus, and water.

A Bit about the Nose of the Matter

I totally agree with the following article from the fragrances of the world web site, The Case for Fragrance Family Loyalty, by Laura Donna, Consumer Fragrance Education.

> "Fine fragrance marketing initiatives and sales training continue to ignore the fundamental tie that binds people to their perfume—the olfactory experience of wearing a favorite scent. The fragrance industry continues to dance around the edges of olfactory marketing, but hasn't gotten religion, investing only half-heartedly in promotional programs based on fragrance families.
>
> Sales training and tools have yet to properly harness the power of The Fragrance Wheel and its ability to predict scents that will inspire loyalty and repeat purchases. New research proves overwhelmingly that women purchase and wear perfume falling into a narrow olfactory range
>
> Isn't it time for the industry to do a better job connecting consumers to scents they will enjoy?" [2]
>
> [That's what I'm talking about!]

 Buzz Notes: Designer perfumes are linked to fashion houses. Chanel No. 5 is the enduring symbol of a designer perfume.[3]

5

Putting It All Together

So now that you've been through Fragrance 101 and know more about the fragrance world, you are ready to spray and play! Hopefully you will be able put it all together and make some amazing discoveries about perfume.

Perhaps the greatest challenge though is dealing with body chemistry. While researching for more information to share with readers, I found the following on the Beauty and the Bath site. It addresses issues for women of all ages. There are also a few concerns for the men, but they just don't seem to have the issues that women do.

> How to Choose the Right Perfume for Your Body Chemistry
>
> You will not know unless you experiment with a variety of fragrances. It is the long-term impression that a fragrance gives you that really counts, not what you think of it at first.

Everyone's skin is different and that is why some fragrances last longer on some people's skin than others. Every individual has their own unique skin chemistry. In fact, your skin chemistry can even change now and again and the changes are not always apparent.

When these changes occur, your fragrance may go from smelling wonderful on you, to not being a very pleasant smell at all. There are a variety of reasons that can contribute to and or cause your skin chemistry to change.

STRESS: The number one reason tends to be stress. If you are feeling a large amount of anxiety it will often effect your heart rate. All of this will factor into a change in your body chemistry and result in your fragrance smelling different.

DIET: What you eat is very closely related to how a fragrance may smell on you.

Your diet can radically change the smell of fragrances on your skin.

For example, too much garlic consumption can cause a slight aroma of garlic to permeate from your skin when you sweat. This aroma may not mix well with your fragrance. Onions as well as other foods that can bring about gas can also alter the aroma of your fragrance.

AGE is something else that can factor into your skin's chemistry. This is because there are a number of significant hormonal changes for men and women. The first change is the shift from child to teen. Puberty can be a hard time on a teenager's body and skin.

PREGNANCY is another event that can cause a major hormonal upheaval. Pregnancy hormones can cause fragrances to smell different to you; a scent you liked before may be something you do not like when expecting.

PERFUME AND MENOPAUSE: Lastly, menopause can bring on changes to your hormones and effect your body chemistry. During this time, your skin can become thinner and drier. Also, testosterone and estrogen levels fluctuate and night sweats often occur.

MEDICATIONS/MEDICAL CONDITIONS: There are also certain medications and even medical conditions that can play a role in how a fragrance will be altered by your body chemistry.

For example, individuals with diabetes will have a harder time finding a fragrance that works well for them. This is due to the fluctuation in their blood sugar levels. As their sugar levels change, so does the scent of the fragrance they are wearing.

Test On Your Skin

Some people have skin that attracts essential oils, this means that their skin may absorb certain oil from a fragrance while other oils dissolve quickly. There is often a lot of testing involved to decide which essential oils work best with your skin chemistry.[1]

Foods That Affect Pheromones

While thinking about this, I found a few facts on eHow about foods that may or may not create the release of human pheromones. I thought this was a good place to insert this information

Pheromones are chemicals secreted by the body that influence the behavior of others of the same species. Each person's pheromones are biologically different, and have a different effect on other people. Scientists believe that human sexual orientation and sexual attraction may be partially based on pheromones.

Humans produce pheromones called aphrodisiacs that affect the sexual behavior of other humans. Though each person produces pheromones with a unique chemical formula, there are certain foods that can affect human pheromones. Does this spark an idea?

Chocolate has long been regarded as a romantic gift. Research indicates that chocolate contains phenylethylamine, a stimulant that causes a sense of excitement and well-being.

Asparagus is high in Vitamin E, which is believed to stimulate sex hormones. In ancient societies, asparagus was considered to be an erotic stimulant because of its phallic shape.

Chili Peppers contain capsaicin, the chemical that adds heat to peppers and other spicy foods. Capsaicin stimulates nerve endings and raises the heart rate, causing the release of endorphins.

Burly Red Wines evoke the scents of leather, tobacco and earth, are said to act as aphrodisiacs. It is believed that the musky bouquet of red wine imitates male hormones.

Celery. The nutrients found in celery are believed to stimulate the pituitary gland, which releases sexual hormones. There is also some evidence to indicate that the scent of celery suggests androstenone, a primary male pheromone. In the Middle Ages, celery was advised as a treatment for impotence.

Oysters. According to legend, Casanova ate oysters everyday, using them to seduce vestal virgins.

Oysters are high in zinc, which is used to produce testosterone.[2]

Here's another article from YouBeauty.com

Sexy Scents That Are Proven to Seduce

If you have ever caught a whiff of someone's perfume as they passed by and thought it to be magical, you are not alone! Psycologists believe that both scent and emotions are processed in the same area of the brain. We find that certain smells can make us feel aroused and stimulated.

I gathered the following thoughts from master perfumer Christine Nagel and Craig Warren, PH D, director of scientific affairs at the Sense of Smell Institute to get their lowdown on which smells seem to hold powerful scents of seduction.

The link between musk and sex is pretty straight forward: Musks replicate the odor secreted from male deer sex glands. According to Nagel, "musk is the most carnal of all fragrance ingredients. It conveys a thin skinned sensuality, and it can easily arouse all the senses. Musk notes were found to have highly sensuous properties. If you're all about primal attraction, these are your go-to fragrances.

VANILLA can get a bad rep for being plain, but it's actually quite the opposite. Long touted as an aphrodisiac, the scent of vanilla can cause arousal and stimulation in both men and women. Nagel says that vanilla may be "soft, almost sweet, but it has a strong, intense, and animalistic facet." As an added bonus, according to Dr. Warren: "Vanilla produces the feeling of happiness universally around the world. Of all the materials that go in fragrances, vanilla is the most liked globally."

PEPPERMINT isn't usually a scent you would associate with sexiness, but according to Nagel, it's an overall "energizing scent, with fresh and fusing notes that release feelings of excitement." Scientific studies have also repeatedly shown that the smell of peppermint has a positive effect on mental stimulation, alertness, and physiological arousal. Dr. Warren agrees that "peppermint is a fragrance that really stimulates and opens all the senses with a secondary effect of making people feel happy." As far as we're concerned, these are all good things when it comes to spending time with a mate.

JASMINE: is the most sensual of all the notes. What makes it unique is that it is a sweet floral note that also has an animalistic characteristic thanks to the presence of indole. What's indole you ask? It's an aromatic compound that also happens to be found in human nether regions. Kinky little flower isn't it? According to Nagel, jasmine exudes a sensual facet." Imagine a bubbly girl next door by day, temptress by night."[3]

 To get your sexy on you might to try these arousing fragrances.

MUSKY: Lancôme Trésor Midnight Rose; Escada Especially Escada.

VANILLA: Boyfriend Eau de Parfum; Burberry Britt and Classic; Estée Lauder Beautiful; Guerlain Oriental Brulant; Marc Jacobs Daisy; Jo Malone London Vanilla and Anise; Marc Jacobs Daisy.

MINTY: Emilio Pucci Vivara Variazioni Verde; Annick Goutal Eau de Sud; Hermè Eau D'Orange Verte.

JASMINE: Bond No. 9 Nuits de NoHo; Bottega Veneta Eau de Parfum; Bulgari Jasmin Noir.

Consider Concentration Strengths

There are several versions of fragrances for both men and women based upon the concentration of essential and fragrance oils. They are not created equal!

Understanding the fragrance strengths takes some of the mystery out of the search for the perfect scent. Also, the mood, the occasion, and the time of year enters into the question of what, where, and when to buy your fragrance.[6]

> ESSENTIAL OILS are natural chemicals that are extracted from the leaves, flowers, stems, roots or bark of plants. They are not true oils, but are the aromatic and volatile essences derived from botanicals.

> FRAGRANCE OILS (also called perfume oils) are usually synthetic; chemists analyze the plants' components and reproduce their chemical compositions.[4]

The Differences of Fragrance Strengths

The concentrations of aromatic ingredients are as follows in ascending order:

1. Splash and aftershave: They have only 1 to 3 percent of aromatic compounds and also define today's popular refreshing body sprays.

2. Eau de cologne: These citrus-type perfumes have about 2 to 6 percent concentrate aromatic compounds.

3. Eau de toilette: These aromatic compounds (5 to 15 percent) have a stronger alcohol base. They are considered as lightly scented perfumes and areoften used as a skin freshener to be applied liberally after bathing.

4. Eau de parfum: This is the second most potent fragrance strength. Although this quality choice has less concentrated essential oils (10 to 20 percent), the scent lasts for a long time. It is not inexpensive but costs much less than the pure perfume.

5. Parfum: This is considered the luxury choice of fragrances. It is the most potent because of its high concentrate of essential oils, usually between 20 and 40 percent. This perfume base lasts longer than lighter versions of a fragrance and is always more expensive.[5]

Thoughts about Not Wearing a Fragrance

If you are a true fragranista like myself, you would want to wear your special fragrance at all times! However; you should actually consider the place, occasion, and overall situation when you decide whether or not to put on your scent. Check out the following article from an eHow contributor

How to Know When Not to Wear Perfume

As much as you love perfume, there are times that wearing perfume should be avoided. Knowing when not to wear perfume is just as important as knowing which perfume to wear at other times.

1. Consider the situation and the impression that you want to leave before spraying on the perfume.
2. Think about the room in which the event will be held. If it will be a small event in a closed room, skip the perfume. It may affect others negatively.
3. Consider the people that you will be with. If any have allergies, don't wear perfume. If you're uncertain, it's better to be safe than sorry.
4. Will you be in a closed car or small space with other people? Most people won't tell you that your perfume bothers them, but more people are affected by scent sensitivities than you think.
5. Consider applying your perfume after you arrive at work if you take public transportation.
6. Leave the perfume off if you have a doctor's or dentist's appointment, and never wear perfume if you are having surgery or X-rays.
7. Skip the perfume at a job interview. You want to be remembered for your skills, not your alluring scent.
8. Don't wear perfume for outdoor picnics or barbecues, especially if they are near gardens. The scent of perfume attracts bees and other insects.[6]

Perfume Ingredient Glossary

I've included here a list of common ingredients found in many perfumes. It is another good start to help identify fragrances.

Perfume Ingredients
An A to Z List of Ingredients Found in Your Favorite Fragrances

Agrumen: An aldehyde (see below) with a characteristic green, musky odor.

Aldehyde: Organic compounds present in many natural materials, that can be synthesized artificially, such as the aliphatic aldehydes used to give sparkle to Chanel No 5.

Amber: A heavy, full bodied, powdery, warm fragrance note. Amber oil comes from the Baltic amber tree.

Ambergris: A sperm whale secretion with a sweet, woody odor. Usually reproduced synthetically.

Ambrett: The oil obtained from ambrette seeds (from the hibiscus) has a musk-like odor. Commonly used as a substitute for true musk.

Amyris: A white-flowering bush or tree found in Haiti and South America. Often used as a less-expensive substitute for sandalwood.

Benzoin: A balsamic resin from the Styrax tree.

Bergamot: The tangy oil expressed from the non-edible bergamot orange, grown mainly in Italy.

Calone: An aroma chemical that adds a "sea breeze" or marine note to fragrances.

Cashmeran: A synthetic aldehyde with a spicy, ambery, musky, floral odor. Used to invoke the velvety smell or "feel" of cashmere.

Castoreum: An animalistic secretion from the Castor beaver, used to impart a leathery aroma to a fragrance. Often reproduced sythetically.

Citron: The zest of this tree's fruit is used to create citrus fragrance notes.

Civet: Musk produced by a gland at the base of the African civet cat's tail. Pure civet is said to have a strong, disagreeable odor, but in small quantities is often used to add depth and warmth to a fragrance.

Clary sage: The oil of this herb smells sweet to bittersweet, with nuances of amber, hay and tobacco.

Coumarin: A commonly used perfume compound that smells like vanilla. Usually derived from the tonka bean (see below), but also found in lavender, sweetgrass and other plants.

Frangipani: A fragrant tropical flower, also known as West Indian jasmine.

Frankincense: A gum resin from a tree found in Arabia and Eastern Africa. Also called Olibanum.

Galbanum: A gum resin that imparts a green smell.

Guaiac Wood: A resinous South American tree whose oil is used in perfumery.

Hedione: An aroma chemical that has a soft, radiant jasmine aroma.

Heliotrope: Flowers of the family heliotropium, which have a strong, sweet vanilla-like fragrance with undertones of almond.

Indole: A chemical compound which smells floral at low concentrations, fecal at high concentrations. Used widely in perfumery.

Iso E Super: An aroma chemical, described as a smooth, woody, amber note with a velvet-like sensation. Used to impart fullness to fragrances.

Jasmine: A flower employed widely in perfumersy. It is the most masculine of the oils and is called "King of the Oils."

Labdanum: An aromatic gum from from the rockrose bush. The sweet woody odor can be used to impart a leather note.

Monoi: Gardenia (tiare) petals macerated in coconut oil. Sometimes called Monoi de Tahiti.

Muguet: French for Lily of the Valley. One of the three most used florals in perfumery. Unlike jasmine and rose, usually synthetically reproduced.

Myrrh: A gum resin produced from a bush found in Arabia and Eastern Africa.

Narcissus: The white flowers of this tree are used extensively in French perfume production.

Neroli: A citrus oil distilled from the blossoms of either the sweet or bitter orange tree. The Italian term for neroli is zagara.

Oakmoss: Derived from a lichen that grows on oak trees. Prized for its aroma, which is heavy and oriental at first, becoming refined and earthy when dried, reminiscent of bark, seashore and foliage.

Opopanax: A herb that grows in the Middle East, North Africa and the Meditarranean, also known as sweet myrrh. The resin produces a scent similar to balsam or lavender.

Orris: Derived from the iris plant. Has a flowery, heavy and woody aroma.

Osmanthus: A flowering tree native to China, valued for its delicate fruity apricot aroma.

Oud (Oudh): Refers to wood from the Agar tree, found mostly in Southeast Asia. The fragrant resin is treasured by perfumers.

Ozone: A modern, synthetic note meant to mimic the smell of fresh air right after a thunderstorm.

Patchouli: A bushy shrub originally from Malaysia and India. Has a musty-sweet, spicy aroma. Often used as a base note.

Rose: One of the main flower notes used in perfumery. (Also known as the "Queen of the Oils.")

Rose de Mai: The traditional name given to Rose Absolute (rose essential oil) produced by solvent then alcohol extraction.

Sandalwood: An oil from the Indian sandal tree. One of the oldest known perfumery ingredients, commonly used as a base note.

Tonka Bean: Derived from a plant native to Brazil. Has an aroma of vanilla with strong hints of cinnamon, cloves and almonds. Used as a less-expensive alternative to vanilla.

Tuberose: A plant with highly-perfumed white flowers, resembling those of a lily.

Vanilla: Derived from the seed pod of the vanilla orchid. Highly fragrant, popular, and expensive to produce.

Vetiver: A grass with heavy, fibrous roots, which are used to distill an oil that smells of moist earth with woody, earthy, leather and smoky undertones. A highly important ingredient in masculine perfumes.

Ylang Ylang: An Asian evergreen tree with fragrant flowers. Used in expensive floral perfumes.[7]

6

Bios of My Fave Perfumers

While researching about the fragrance world, I especially enjoyed learning about the men and women whose creativity inspired its modernization. I've chosen four people who have wonderful stories worth sharing and who became legends in their own time.

My most favorite success story is about Gabrielle Chanel, known as Coco. She was a nonconformist who followed her dreams and passion to create understated elegance in both the worlds of fashion and fragrance.

Coco launched her first fragrance in 1920s, which was also the first perfume that featured its designer's name: Chanel.

Another favorite beauty icon was derived from early childhood recollections of my own wonderful mother and her Estée Lauder fragrance. My oldest son commented once that "Mama Edie was not afraid of perfume!"

Third on my list of faves is Thierry Mugler. His work challenges the modern world through his imagination, excellence, and creativity. He is especially known for his fragrance known as "Angel", the first oriental gourmand perfume.

And last, but certainly not least, Michael Edwards! He is known as the "perfume experts' expert," and I found his website to be the best reference source available. Also, his fragrance wheel inspired me to create my own fragrance chart, which gives even greater solidarity to my "fragranista theory."

About Coco Chanel

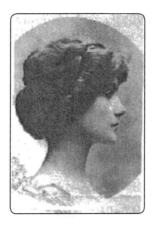

Perfume is the unseen, unforgettable, ultimate accessory of fashion…that heralds your arrival and prolongs your departure. (Coco Chanel)

Fashion designer Gabrielle "Coco" Chanel was born August 19, 1883, in Saumur, France. She is famous for her timeless designs, trademark suits, little black dresses and of course, her fabulous fragrances. She had a brief career as a singer before opening her first clothes shop in 1910. In the 1920s, she launched her first perfume and introduced the Chanel suit and the little black dress.

Her early years, however, were anything but glamorous. After her mother's death, Chanel was put in an orphanage by her father who worked as a peddler. She was raised by nuns who taught her how to sew—a skill that would lead to her life's work. Her nickname came from another occupation entirely.

During her brief career as a singer, Chanel performed in clubs in Vichy and Moulins where she was called "Coco." Some say that the name comes from one of the songs she used to sing, and Chanel herself said that it was a "shortened version of cocotte, the French word for 'kept woman.'"

Coco Chanel created timeless designs that are still popular today. She herself became a much revered style icon known for her simple yet sophisticated outfits paired with great accessories, such as several strands of pearls. As Chanel once said, "luxury must be comfortable, otherwise it is not luxury."

Fashion Pioneer

Around the age of 20, Chanel became involved with Etienne Balsan who offered to help her start a millinery business in Paris. She soon left him for one of his even wealthier friends, Arthur "Boy" Capel. Both men were instrumental in Chanel's first fashion venture.

Opening her first shop on Paris's Rue Cambon in 1910, Chanel started out selling hats. She later added stores in Deauville and Biarritz and began making clothes. Her first taste of clothing success came from a dress she fashioned out of an old jersey on a chilly day. In response to the many people who asked about where she got the dress, she offered to make one for them. "My fortune is built on that old jersey that I'd put on because it was cold in Deauville," she once told author Paul Morand.

In the 1920s, Chanel took her thriving business to new heights. She launched her first perfume, Chanel No. 5, which would later become the single most recognized women's fragrance in the world. It was also the first perfume to feature a designer's name. Another 1920s revolutionary design was Chanel's little black dress. She took a color once associated with mourning and showed just how chic it could be for evening wear. In addition to fashion, Chanel was a popular figure in the Paris literary and artistic worlds. She designed costumes for the Ballets Russes and for Jean Cocteau's play Orphée, and count Cocteau and artist Pablo.

In 1925, she introduced the now legendary Chanel suit with collarless jacket and well-fitted skirt. Her designs were revolutionary for the time—borrowing elements of men's wear and emphasizing comfort over the constraints of then-popular fashions. She helped women say good-bye to the days of corsets and other confining garments.

Legacy

Coco Chanel died on January 10, 1971, at her apartment in the Hotel Ritz. She never married, having once said, "I never wanted to weigh more heavily on a man than a bird." Hundreds crowded together at the Church of the Madeleine to bid farewell to the fashion icon. In tribute, many of the mourners wore Chanel suits.

A little more than a decade after her death, designer Karl Lagerfeld took the reins at her company to continue the Chanel legacy. Today her namesake company continues to thrive and is believed to generate hundreds of millions in sales each year.

In addition to the longevity of her designs, Chanel's life story continues to captivate people's attention. There have been several biographies of the fashion revolutionary, including Chanel and Her World (2005) written by her friend Edmonde Charles-Roux.

In the recent television biopic, Coco Chanel (2008), Shirley MacLaine starred as the famous designer around the time of her 1954 career resurrection. The actress had long been interested in playing Chanel. "What's wonderful about her is she's not a straightforward, easy woman to understand."

Perfume History

In 1921 Coco Chanel debuted her first perfume, which would later become the single most recognized women's fragrance in the world: Chanel No. 5. In 1955 she introduced her first-ever men's scent, Pour Monsieur. After her death, more fragrances would emerge: Cristalle au de toilette and for men, Antaeus.

In 1981 Karl Lagerfeld became Artistic Director of Chanel Fashion and with him came even more successful scents. In 1984 he launched Coco, a fragrance homage to the late iconic designer. With the immense success of the female scent Allure in 1996 , he created a version for men. That cologne is appropriately named Allure Homme. The latest perfume to make its debut is Chance.

Today Chanel is one of the few luxury houses to have its own in-house creator-composer, Jacques Polge. He is also known as and called 'THE nose!' in the world of fragrances. [1]

—∿—

About Estée Lauder

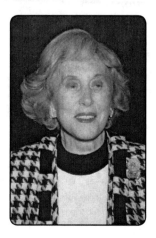

When I began in the industry, fragrance was a luxury, not a tool for success. I am proud to think that I had something to do with encouraging the American woman to wear perfume every day of the week. (Estée Lauder)

Estée Lauder is one of the wealthiest self-made women in America. Examine the public and private life of the woman who built her cosmetics empire on the dream of every woman: to feel beautiful.

With the introduction of her first fragrance, Youth-Dew in 1953, EstéeLauder invited women to think about fragrance in a completely different way. She convinced them to buy fragrance for themselves and to use it lavishly rather than save and to use it for special occasions.

With each new fragrance she developed, Mrs. Lauder took risks, challenging traditional rules of fragrance development. She established new standards of creativity and new fragrance categories, soon to be studied and imitated by others.

As a teenager, Estée was "caught up with American glamour and dreamed of being a skin specialist and making women beautiful.

Early years

Josephine Esther Mentzer, daughter of immigrants, lived above her father's hardware store. She started her enterprise by selling skin creams concocted by her uncle, a chemist, in beauty shops, beach clubs and resorts.

She met Joseph Lauter when she was in her early 20s and they married on 15 January 1930. Their surname later changed to Lauder and Josephine dropped her first name when naming her cosmetics brand.

Their son Leonard was born on 19 March 1933 and the couple separated in 1939 when she moved to Florida. However, they remarried in 1942 and had a second son called Ronald. They stayed married until Joseph's death in 1982.

Early career

Lauder established the Estée Lauder company in 1935 and her first foray into commercial success occurred after Florence Morris, the owner of the House of Ash Blondes salon, asked Lauder how she got such perfect skin. She returned to the salon with her uncle's creams and showed customers how to use them. Lauder was then asked to sell them at the establishment.

Buzz Note: Estée Lauder built her cosmetic empire on the dream of every woman: to feel beautiful.

In 1948, she persuaded the bosses of New York City department stores to give her counter space at Saks Fifth Avenue. Once in that space, she utilized a personal selling approach that proved as potent as the promise of her skin regimens and perfumes. Even after 40 years in business, Estée Lauder would attend every launch of a new cosmetics counter or shop.

She would give her famous friends and acquaintances small samples of her products for their handbags; she wanted her brand in the hands of people who were known for having "the best." One person that Lauder sent her products to was the actress and later Princess of Monaco, Grace Kelly.

Estée Lauder loved to hold large dinner parties. She enjoyed "beautiful people," celebrities, the rich and famous, and could invite them to dine with her at a table that could seat 30 without extensions.

Fragrance Launch

In 1953, Lauder introduced her first fragrance, Youth Dew, a bath oil that doubled as a perfume. Instead of using their French perfumes by the drop behind each ear, women were using Youth Dew by the bottle in their bath water.

In the first year, Youth Dew sold fifty thousand. By 1984, the figure had jumped to 150 million.

She was the subject of a TV documentary in 1985 called 'Estée Lauder: The Sweet Smell of Success' in which she explained that she had never worked a day in her life without selling.

Lauder and both her sons are billionaires, with sales going up every year, as Estée Lauder products remain one of the most popular cosmetics lines. The brand is now recognized in over 120 countries.

She died of cardiopulmonary arrest on 26 April 2004. She was aged at least 95. Today Estée Lauder continues to be at the forefront of creative fragrance development with a portfolio of 28 innovative fragrances.

Beautiful, Estée Lauder's classic lush floral, is the number one best-selling fragrance in the United States and a fragrance favorite for millions of women for over 25 years.[2]

—∽—

About Thierry Mugler

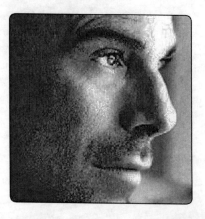

Thierry Mugler is an instinctive designer who never looks for inspiration and has been referred to as "the prophet of futurism." Fashion Model Directory (FMD)[3]

Mugler was born in Strasbourg, France on 21 December 1948. He began ballet lessons at age nine but his passion led him to focus more on drawing than on school. At the age of 14, he began taking classes in interior design at the Strasbourg School of Decorative Art. About the same time he joined the ballet corps for the Rhin Opera (Opéra national du Rin).[4]

He took great interest in the costume design and so began the passion for clothing. He began to travel the world and study fashion at the age of 24. He became quite well known from the success of both women and men's clothing lines that were both sophisticated and urban.

His career path led him to design costumes and help create and direct short films, musical videos, and also stage and movie performances. He also created the famous black dress worn by Demi Moore in the 1993 movie, 'Indecent Proposal.'[5]

As with many successful designers and celebrities he moved his name and creativity into the fragrance world. In 1992 he launched "Angel," the first oriental gourmand fragrance that combines chocolate and praline sweetness with patchouli which is bottled as a blue liquid in a glass refillable star.

He has a fascination with the heavens and his signature star is a constant design feature to his fragrance line.

Early career

At the age of 24, Mugler decided to travel the world and left Strasbourg to go live in Paris. He began designing clothes for a small, trendy Parisian boutique by the name of "Gudule." At 26, Mugler, who was working as a freelance designer, began to work for a variety of large ready-to-wear fashion houses in Paris, Milan, London and Barcelona.

In 1973 Mugler created his first personal collection called "Café de Paris." The style of the collection was both sophisticated and urban. Melka Tréanton, a powerful fashion editor, helped launched his career. In 1976, she asked him to show his work in Tokyo, for an event organized by Shiseido. In 1978 he opened his first Paris boutique at the place des Victoires.

At the same time, Thierry Mugler launched a fashion collection for men. For this collection, he reworked classical masculinity giving it a definitively modern style. A clean, precise, structured cut which outlined a highly-recognizable silhouette: prominent shoulders, both "anatomical and classic," for a dynamic and slender look.

During the 1980s and 1990s Thierry Mugler had become an internationally recognized designer and his collections garnered much commercial success. At the request of the Chambre Syndicale de la Haute Couture, he completed his first haute couture collection in 1992. [6]

Fragrances

Thierry Mugler's first perfume appeared in 1992 and was called Angel. "Angel" opened a new olfactory trend with its combination of praline and chocolate-derived sweetness mixed with a strong accent of patchouli. Angel was the first oriental gourmand perfume and comes in an unprecedented color for a women's fragrance: blue.

The Angel bottle, a complicated design in the shape of a faceted star, was created by the Brosse Master Glassmakers. Today, more than thirteen engraved and numbered Limited Edition stars have been successively created for several holiday seasons.

Other perfumes have been developed to enrich the brand's fragrance universe, including three major fragrances: A*Men, Mugler Cologne and Alien.

In 2005, Alien was created, the second major Thierry Mugler fragrance, inspired by a solar world, filled with hope, serenity and light. Also in 2005, Thierry Mugler launched the "Thierry Mugler Perfume Workshops" which are open to the general public and led by specialists of the perfumery and oenology world. The goal of these workshops is to convey the art and know-how of the industry along with the craftsmanship of making perfume. [7]

Other Creations

In 2006, Thierry Mugler completed a project for the launch of Tom Tykwer's film "Perfume." In collaboration with the IFF company, Thierry Mugler created a box set of fifteen compositions.

During 2007, still following the metamorphosis theme, Mugler launched Mirror, Mirror, a collection of five fragrances, created as "perfume-trickery" to "enhance one's presence."

Finally, on 8 March 2010, Thierry Mugler launched the site womanity.com, a virtual space for expression which asks visitors to share their vision on what it means to be a woman today. The site corresponded to Womanity, the newest fragrance by the house of Mugler which was released at the same time.

According to popular descriptions, "It evokes the emotion of tender childhood memories together with a sense of dreamlike infinity. Angel, which launched a new fragrance category called the "oriental gourmands," seduces us with angelic flavors found deep within the heart of our memories, as well as sensual and passionate notes. [8]

About Michael Edwards

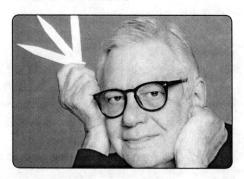

"A great perfume is a work of art. It is silent poetry (that) can lift our days, enrich our nights and create the milestones of our memories. Fragrance is liquid emotion." (Michael Edwards)

Michael Edwards, is known as the "perfume experts' expert." He has been a major influence in the fragrance industry over the past thirty years, and his annual fragrance guide, *Fragrances of the World*, now celebrates its thirty-first edition.

What started in 1983 as a simple guide for retailers, listing 323 fragrances, has grown into a comprehensive classification system of fragrances worldwide. Its purpose is to make fragrance selection an exciting journey rather than a difficult chore. It is now universally regarded as the fragrance 'bible' by perfumers, industry professionals, journalists and fragrance connoisseurs, this year classifying over 8,000 fragrances including 1,200 of new releases.

It is the only guide that maintains its independence, accepting no advertising or fees for its listings. The rigorous classification methodology whereby the fragrance gets assigned to a particular family cannot be understated–Michael and his team personally test every fragrance and then cross-check their findings with the perfumers to ensure the accuracy of the listings.

Fragrance Wheel

Edwards also created the Fragrance Wheel in 1983. The families, on which the Wheel is based, hold the key to people's likes and dislikes because each family has a characteristic scent whose personality is reflected in its fragrance.

The Fragrance Wheel maps out the connections among groups of scents. It includes the three major families defined by perfumers—Floral, Oriental, Woody, as well as a fourth one, the Fresh, which was introduced by Edwards. "It makes selecting the right perfume an exciting process of discovery." [As of yet, it] is the only complete, accurate and industry respected fragrance classification system.

Perfume Legends

Michael's book, Perfume Legends: French Feminine Fragrances, published in 1998, opened up the secret world of perfumery and instantly became a cult classic given its in depth historical research. For the first time, perfumers spoke of their work and the sources of their inspiration.

Since his early days in Paris, Edwards has been impressed and fascinated by the work of fragrance creators and yet surprised by the lack of public knowledge about their work. Through his revealing stories of the greatest fragrances ever created, he offers a tribute to perfumers and provides a glimpse into the complex and intricate process of fragrance creation.

In 2005 Michael went on to introduce Fragrances of the World.Info–the world's only fragrance database that sorts and cross-references over 16,000 fragrances by classifications, pyramid and accord notes, perfumers and bottle designers, bottle images, house and corporate groups, gender, country, and year of launch.

The online database offers such a wealthy source of information that the industry recognized Michael twice with the highly prestigious FiFi award for Technological Breakthrough

A self-proclaimed gypsy, Michael divides his time among Sydney, Paris and New York in order to stay abreast of the market and to keep industry in touch with the latest developments.

As Edwards chooses to cover new fragrance markets—Latin America, Middle East and Asia—the scope of his work continues to expand, yet he is undaunted. After all, every new fragrance offers a new experience, a new memory, a new story.[9]

I end chapter 6 with this passage from Michael Edward's wonderful book, *Perfume Legends: French Feminine Fragrances.*

> "First you learn to smell," says Roja Dove. "You learn the smell of your mother, the scent of home. Then, as you grow up, you start to learn about fragrances. When you become a little bit older, you learn about fine French fragrances, and then, hopefully, you learn about the Guerlain fragrances. When in the end, you appreciate L'Heure Bleu, then you know that you really love perfume."

As of yet I have not discovered L'Heure Bleu, but I definitely intend to do so.

7

One Hundred Fragrance Tips

Q&A

Over the years, I have repeatedly heard many of the same questions. Since there are no dumb questions, I decided to research them and include the best answers I could find from a few top professionals and more from the eHow site.

Follow fashion and beauty blog sites for more answers to your questions. Other readers love to interact with their discoveries and opinions. You just might run across some great information that you did not already know!

36 Q&As from Michael Edwards's Fragrances of the World Site

Q1: How many different fragrances can I try without confusing my sense of smell?

A: Three. Although you will find your sense of smell tires more quickly from similar fragrances than fragrances of very different character, you risk confusing your sense if you test more than three different scents at one time.

Q2: How can I make my fragrance last longer?

A: The secret to long-lasting fragrance is 'fragrance layering'. Build up layers of scent on the skin by using different forms of the same fragrance—perfumed soap, bath oil or gel, body lotion or cream, dusting powder and eau de toilette. Each reinforces the impact of the other to quadruple the life of your favourite scent. Layering, or "fragrance dressing" as it's sometimes called, is also a clever way to wear a fragrance that's too overpowering for daytime use.

Q3: How should I store my perfume?

A: Keep your fragrances in a cool, dry place away from direct sunlight and heat sources (such as radiators). Extreme heat or cold will upset the delicate balance of the oils and change their scent. Once a bottle of perfume is opened, use it. A spray lets in less air and evaporates slower than a bottle with a cap but even the finest essence fades with time. If you prefer one fragrance in winter and another in the summer, you'll extend their life between seasons if you store the bottle in the vegetable crisper of the refrigerator.

Q4: Is perfume an aphrodisiac?

A: Scent can certainly make you feel sexier but there is no scientific evidence to suggest that fragrance is actually an aphrodisiac. Smell is obviously linked to our sexuality and some experts believe that hormones released from glands in the groin and armpit act as powerful sexual attractants in the way that pheromones released by animals do. The sense of confidence the right perfume can give, plus the attractive chemical cocktail it helps create, can certainly be a great turn-on.

Q5: Do women have a keener sense of smell than men?

A: "Yes," says Richard L. Doty, Director of the Smell and Taste Centre at the University of Pennsylvania, USA. But, he adds, the male/female differences may well be cultural–or hormonal. Women in our society tend to use their sense of smell more often than men. They are encouraged to take an interest in cooking, flowers and fragrance.

A woman's sense of smell also fluctuates more than a man's, which makes her more aware of fragrances and odours. These fluctuations seem to be influenced by the release of certain hormones during the menstrual cycle. Oestrogen increases smell acuity in the first half of the month, and again in the early months of pregnancy, while progesterone decreases the ability to smell in the last half.

Q6: Why do we wear (and love) fragrance so much?

A: Because it helps us feel good about ourselves and others. Recent psychological tests show that people who use fragrance regularly have a more positive attitude toward socializing and may be more socially skilled than those who seldom or never wear it. It was generally found that people who believe that others think they smell good have more confidence.

Q7: Why do I hate some fragrances and love others?

A: Because we all are programmed to like certain smells and dislike others. Our response to odor and fragrance, say scientists, is partly learned and partly genetic. We are born with definite likes and dislikes, as well as sensitivity to certain smells. Very early on, experience starts modifying and adding to them and we build up a complex "smell bank" of memories and associations. All this stored information determines whether or not we like a fragrance.

Q8: Will my taste in perfume change as I get older?

A: Probably. As you grow older and the way you feel about yourself changes, the kind of fragrance you choose will change too. (Typically) teens... wear light, gentle scents. In your late teens and early twenties, you'll often choose a fragrance because you identify with its image. As your sense of confidence develops, you tend to choose a fragrance that expresses your individual style, your personal taste.

Q9: When shouldn't I wear perfume?

A: In the sun. Fragrance tends to react with ultraviolet light, irritating the skin and often causing skin discoloration. There are, however, some specially formulated alcohol-free, safe to wear in summer.

Q10: What should I do if I develop an allergy to a perfume?

A: If you feel a wave of nausea, take a deep breath of fresh air. Breathe deeply for a few minutes, blowing through your nose to clear the nasal passages.

If your skin is red and itchy, splash the area with cold water for a few minutes and pat dry. Some areas such as the neck are more sensitive than others, so if the reaction is only mild, you could try the fragrance on a less sensitive part of the body.

Safer pulse points are: below the ears and knees, at the bend of the elbow, on the bosom and around wrists. If the fragrance still irritates your skin, but you love it so much that you want to keep wearing it, here's the answer: spray a cotton ball, let dry and tuck it into your bra.

Finding the Right Fragrance

Q11: How do the fragrance families help me choose the right perfume?

A: Because our sense of smell is so emotional, we assume that fragrances are confusing, a jumble of different perfumes with no rhyme or reason.

It's not true. When you classify the fragrances you have worn, you'll probably find that they fall mostly into just two or three families. Once you know the families you especially like, the Fragrance Manual will show you which other fragrances fall into the same family.

Q12: How do I select a fragrance as a gift for a woman?

A: One sure way is find out which fragrances she especially likes, the names of her favorite perfumes. Once you know those magic names, an informed consultant will be able to help you select another fragrance from the same family or families of fragrance that she especially likes.

If you don't know the names of her favorite fragrances, ask a consultant for advice. Describe the lady for whom you're buying the gift–not her hair colour (will it be the same next week?) nor her age (we all know women who're old at 20, others who are vibrant at 70), but her style of dress, her personality, her activities. Ask the consultant to suggest three fragrances, just three, never more. Test their scents on testing papers. Take your time. Which fragrance 'talks' to you? Try not to be logical. Relax. Let your instinct take over. Nine times out of ten, you'll find that your nose will select the perfect match.

How to Test a Fragrance

Q13: What is the correct way to try a fragrance?

A: Apply a few drops or the lightest spray to your wrist or the back of your hand. Don't just sniff a flacon because perfume comes to life only on your skin. Wait a few moments. Give the fragrance time to bloom on your skin, to let the notes 'talk' to you.

Q14: When testing a fragrance which concentration should I use?

A: Lighter fragrance concentrations such as eaux de toilette or colognes, because they dry and develop quickly.

Q15: What's the best way to try on several fragrances?

A: Apply the first fragrance to one wrist and wait a few minutes. Apply the second to the other wrist and a third fragrance to the inside of the elbow. Remember, three is the maximum number of fragrances you should try on at once. Any more and your nose is likely to become confused.

Q16: Where else can I spray perfume, apart from my skin?

A: Try the lightest spray through damp hair before you blow dry, or mist your hairbrush and comb with fragrance before use. Perhaps a touch of perfume on your handkerchief. A spray of essence on padded hangers. Add a few drops of perfume to the water in a steam iron to lace clothes with fragrance, or rinse lingerie in scented water.

Q17: How long will an opened bottle of perfume last?

A: Depending on the fragrance, from six to 18 months, if stored correctly. Once a bottle of fragrance has been opened it should be used because all fragrance deteriorates with time: light, citrus-based perfumes in as little as six months; floral scents in about a year and a half.

Q18: How can I tell if a perfume has gone off?

A: When its color has changed, when it seems thicker or when the initial notes seem sour, almost "off."

Q19: What packaging helps keep perfume the longest?

A: Spray forms rather than regular bottles, because an atomizer admits less air than a bottle with a screw-on cap, limits contamination and slows down the evaporation of the perfume.

Psychological Effects

Q20: Can fragrance change my mood?

A: Yes! One of the most remarkable properties of fragrance is the way it instantly affects our emotions. Studies have shown that fragrances can stimulate or calm us, encourage a good mood or bad, shape positive or negative memories and induce sweet dreams.

Aromatherapy–the art of healing with fragrant essential oils–is based on the idea that aroma has the power to affect mood.

In a recent study, peppermint and lily of the valley were found to increase alertness at work. One Tokyo company pipes peppermint into the office to improve productivity. Another company sends different fragrances through the air conditioning system to enhance staff productivity. A whiff of citrus helps get the day off to a good start. An unobtrusive floral fragrance aids concentration in mid-morning and afternoon. A touch of cedar seems to relieve tiredness during the lunch break and in the late afternoon.

Q21: Do certain personality types like different types of scent?

A: Yes. We buy fragrances not only because we like their smell but also because they reflect our personality.

According to studies carried out by the psychologist and sociologist Dr Joachim Mensing of the Research Institute for Applied Aesthetics in Freiburg, Germany, "extroverts" look for stimulation from the environment and tend to find fresh, green fragrances activating. "Introverts," who prefer less stimulation, find Orientals harmonious, while emotionally ambivalent people–dreamers–prefer floral, powdery scents.

But, a word of caution: this work was researched in Germany, on a fairly small sample of people.

Q22: Why is scent so sexy?

A: "The nose may really be a sexual organ–it may be more closely related to sexual response than vision," suggests American researcher, Michael Shipley. Clearly, the sheer confidence and heightened sensuality produced by the right fragrance makes us more receptive to sexual feelings and more attractive to others.

Q23: Why does a perfume smell wonderful on a friend but not on me?

A: Because each of us has our own "scent print" that will influence the development of a perfume. This odor-identity is the sum total of our genes, our skin chemistry, diet, medication intake, stress level and, probably the most important factor of all, the temperature of our skin.

It's not as simple as saying that fragrances react differently on different people because of their 'body chemistry'. The warmth of our skin is critical. Some people have more pores per centimeter than others, or more layers of fat in their skin. These and other factors affect the warmth of skin, which in turn influences the scent of a fragrance.

Q24: I've been wearing the same fragrance for years, so why does it seem so different now?

A: Probably because your personal chemistry and body temperature have changed slightly. Perhaps you are on a low-fat diet or taking some new medication. Have you changed your brand of contraceptive pill? Are you pregnant? Are you exercising more frequently? Has your skin become drier? Are you using more moisturizer?

Fragrance formulae rarely change but diet or medication changes produce new chemicals that come through the pores and can change the fragrance balance on your skin.

Q25: Is it true that fragrance reacts differently on blondes, brunettes and redheads?

A: Probably. True blondes often have a dry skin that lacks the oils needed to hold scent. As a result, fragrances evaporate more rapidly from their skin.

Brunettes, on the other hand, usually have skin that holds fragrance well because it is much richer in natural oils.

True redheads generally have skin that's fair and delicate, characterised by fine pores and a slightly higher body temperature. Their skin releases the true notes of most fragrances but its warmth tends to make fragrances fade quite quickly.

Q26: Can dieting affect the amount of fragrance I need to apply?

A: Yes. If you're on a low-fat diet, the oil levels in your skin tend to be lower so you may find that your fragrance does not seem to last as long.

Q27: Is it true that antibiotics may change my fragrance?

A: Yes. Firstly, because many antibiotics change the smell of your skin. Secondly, because their action decimates the bacteria on your skin, which, in turn blend with your skin oils to produce a fragrance that is distinctive to you.

Men's Cologne

Q28: Are certain men's fragrances also best for certain seasons?

A: Yes. As with women's fragrance, heavier notes are best in the colder months; lighter fragrances are more suited to summer weather. If you like to wear the more potent, heavier fragrances year round, consider using the lighter aftershave version as a body cologne in warmer weather.

Q29: Is there a golden rule when it comes to men and men's fragrance?

A: "Less is more." Fragrance is always more potent than one imagines. A man often uses a fragrance more liberally than a woman would because his sense of smell tends not to be as acute. Also, men become used to splashing on an aftershave and forget that a cologne or an eau de toilette has a more concentrated, far more potent fragrance.

Q30: I use an electric razor? Should I still use an aftershave?

A: Yes. Shaving is shaving. An electric razor is just as likely to irritate skin, so it makes sense to use an aftershave to soothe sensitive patches, to heal surface nicks. For drier skins, use an aftershave balm or moisturizer.

Q31: Should I use a cologne or an eau de toilette on my face?

A: Neither. Never. Ever. They can be murder to a man's skin. The act of shaving, the daily pruning of some 16,000 whiskers, scrapes away layers of dead skin cells to expose new skin that is unprotected and very sensitive. A cologne or eau de toilette will create `shaving shock' if splashed onto freshly shaved skin. Its high alcohol content will burn and dry the new, raw skin. Use an aftershave or a balm on your face and reserve the cologne or eau de toilette for your body.

Q32: Can I revive the fragrance of an aftershave or cologne?

A: Yes. Splash just a little water on your face, or on the spots where you originally applied the fragrance. The water will mix with your skin oils and revive the fragrance for a while.

Q33: Will the same aftershave smell differently on different men?

A: Yes, because each man's body chemistry and skin type is a little different. The logic is this: fragrance molecules are oil-soluble, so the oilier the skin, the slower the fragrance release and the longer the scent will last.

Tip 34: Men with oily skins should keep away from heavy, oriental notes. Choose light, crisp fragrances: Citrus and Green notes or the Fresh/ Crisp interpretations of Florals, Orientals, Woody notes or Aromatic Fougère fragrances.

Tip 35: Men with a dry skin will probably need a more potent, richer fragrance to hold the notes. Choose any rich interpretations from the Fragrance Manual or select from the Soft Oriental, Oriental or Woody Oriental families.

Tip 36: Generally, men with blond hair and blue eyes will tend to have dry skin. The darker the skin, the browner the eyes, the more likely a man's skin will be oily, the longer it will hold a fragrance.[1]

Tips from eHow.com

How to Wear Perfume

Tip 37: A brief warning. Exercise caution if applying fragrance to clothing. The aromatic chemicals in perfume can stain clothing and cause spotting and fading.

Tip 38: Apply perfume to the pulse points of the wrists and throat. A couple of spritzes from about 6 inches away should moisten the skin slightly. Do not over-apply thinking that the scent should stay strong all day long. Subtly is the key to proper application.

Tip 39: Restrain from spraying more perfume periodically throughout the day. The nose becomes desensitized to fragrances and an individual will not be able to smell their own scent while others still can.

Tip 40: Spray some cologne on the nape of the neck and shoulder for intimate moments. A woman's partner will be pleasantly surprised by a hint of perfume along the collar bone or on the lower back. The scent should only be as strong as a single flower and not overpowering.

Tip 41: Add just a hint of another fragrance to a different area of the body, such as the back or lower legs. This nearly imperceptible interchange of fragrances will register subconsciously with others and cause them to take notice

Tip 42: For a light scent, pump a few sprays of perfume in front of you and walk through the mist to catch the odor on your clothes and hair.

Tip 43: Don't store perfume in the refrigerator or in the bathroom medicine cabinet. The extreme cold is just as damaging to the scent as extreme heat. [Refer back to Q-3].[2]

More eHow Tips

How to Make Perfume Last Longer

Tip 45: Whether floral, musky or citrusy, perfume is a well-chosen accessory that when worn often enough can become a "signature scent."

Tip 46: Pick your potion. Perfume makers say that pure perfume oils and perfumes made with a high concentration of essential oils last longer than perfumes diluted with ethyl alcohol, water or other substances. In general, the lower concentration of fillers involved, the longer the fragrance lasts.

Tip 47: Perfume extract and eau de parfum have the highest concentration of perfume oil; eau de toilette and eau de cologne have the lowest.

Tip 48: Manufacturers estimate that the scent of a perfume or parfum can last up to six hours, depending on a wearer's body chemistry; the scent from eau de toilette and eau de cologne can wear off after about two to four hours.

Tip 49: When applying, consider warmth and moisture. Perfume reacts well to body temperature, so you'll smell the scent strongest when you apply it to your pulse points—-inside the wrists, behind the ears, behind the knees, the back of the neck, in the cleavage.

Tip 50: Perfume also clings better to skin that is naturally oily or moist from a shower because of the evaporating properties of the alcohol mixed with many scents. This is why manufacturers make not only perfume but scented body wash, lotion and powder to match.

Tip 51: Applying a scent in layers—-for instance, using scented body wash followed by lotion and cologne—-will make the scent linger. If you don't want to layer your scent, at least apply perfume or cologne to freshly moisturized skin before you dress.

Tip 52: Store perfume carefully. Manufacturers estimate that the shelf life of a perfume is about three to five years, depending on its ingredients and storage.

Tip 53: Extreme light or heat is poison to perfume, because it can change the perfume's composition or color.

Tip 54: Although the bottles look beautiful arranged in on a bedroom vanity, the best storage place for perfume is tucked in its original box and kept at room temperature—-perhaps in a sock or underwear drawer.

Tip 55: A dark or opaque bottle will keep the scent longer than a clear one.

Tip 56: Cap the bottle tightly, if it's not a spray, to avoid evaporation.

Tip 57: When the perfume smells odd or changes color or consistency, toss it.[3]

Skin-Related Questions

Q-58: You've found the perfect scent at an affordable price, but whenever you wear it, it's gone within a few hours. Why does that happen?

A: Maintain healthy skin to enhance perfume.

Tip: 59: Healthy skin is key to the successful use of beauty products. First, ensure that your skin is thoroughly washed prior to applying perfume.

Tip 60: Evaluate yourself for any particular skin or body issues that may cause you to have a strong body odor. If you use perfume to mask body odor, it will not last as long, and eventually your body odor will overpower the perfume.

Tip 61: If you have any skin or body issues that could be disrupting the use of your perfume, address them by seeking professional help or using appropriate products before applying perfume.

Tip 62: Ensure that you are not using perfume in place of a deodorant or antiperspirant. Even deodorants with a light smell will not mask your perfume, but instead enhance it. The deodorant will take away any odor from sweat, allowing your perfume to gracefully scent the remainder of your body.

Tip 63: Ensure that you have no open irritations or sores on your body before applying perfume, as the combination of perfume and bodily fluids can combine to create unpleasant odors.

Provide Moisture to Prolong Perfume

Tip 64: Provide moisture to prolong perfume because it lasts longer in a moist environment. Before applying perfume, first evaluate the state of your skin-is it dry and flaky, or moist and healthy?

Tip 65: If your skin is dry, apply a moisturizer to help bring fluids to your skin. Consider buying a lotion that is the same scent as your perfume.

Tip 66: Allow the moisturizer to be fully absorbed by your skin before applying perfume.

Tip 67: Identify your pressure points, and ensure that they have already been moisturized. The most common areas to spritz with perfume are your wrists, your neck and behind your knees.

Tip 68: Spray perfume across your body, making sure to cover your pressure points for maximum staying power.[4]

A Bit about Pheromones

(This section gets a bit scientific, but read on if you wish to enlighten yourself.)

Q69: What in the world is a pheromone?

A: According to *Merriam Webster*, a pheromone is "a chemical substance that is usually produced by an animal and serves especially as a stimulus to other individuals of the same species for one or more behavioral responses."

Q70: Do Pheromones Play a Role in Our Sex Lives?

A: Article from the Scientific American site:

"Scientists have long debated whether...sexual attraction is literally in the air, in the form of chemicals called pheromones. Creatures from mice to moths send out these chemical signals to entice mates. And if advertisements about pheromone-laden fragrances are to be believed, one might conclude that humans also exchange molecular come-hithers."

Q71: Is human pheromonal attraction fact or fiction?

A: Based on scientific study, the jury is still "out" on this one. For more information on current studies read more of the above cited article by Adam Hadhazy from scientificamerican.com.

A Bit More about Pheromones

Tip 72: Humans: Body Odor

While humans are highly dependent upon visual cues, when in close proximity smells also play a big role in sociosexual behaviors.

Tip 73: Human Pheromones

There is an inherent difficulty in studying human pheromones because of the need for cleanliness and odorlessness in human participants. The focus of the experiments on human pheromones has been on three classes of putative pheromones: axillary steroids, vaginal aliphatic acids, and stimulators of the vomeronasal organ.[6]

Q74: What are Axillary Steroids

A: There are three axillary steroids that have been described as human pheromones: androstenone, androstenol, and androstandienone. The axillary steroids are produced by the testes, ovaries, apocrine glands and adrenal glands. These chemicals are not biologically active until puberty when the sex steroids influence their activity. This change in activity associated with puberty is some of the best evidence that our species do communicate through odors.[7]

Q75: What are Stimulators of the Vomeronasal Organ?

A: The human vomeronasal organ has epithelia (layers of cells that may be able to serve as a chemical sensory organ; however, the genes that encode the VNO receptors are nonfunctional pseudogenes in humans. Also, while there are sensory neurons in the human VNO there seem to be no connections between the VNO and the central nervous system. The associated olfactory bulb is present in the fetus but regresses and vanishes in the adult brain. There have been some reports that the human VNO does function, but only responds to hormones in a "sex-specific manner." There also has been pheromone receptor genes found in olfactory mucosa. Unfortunately, there have been no experiments that compare people lacking the VNO and people that have it. It is still disputed on whether the chemicals are reaching the brain through the VNO or other tissues.[8]

Q76: Find Anything Less Scientific about Pheromones?

A: Yes! My search found a site that is more than a bit less scientific. The author signs off simply as Greg, from: truth-about-pheromones.com.[9] I liked his story about his personal search and experiments to find some truth about pheromones.

Q77: What Did Greg Find?

A: He is confident that 'sprays and cologne do not work' but hormone releasers do. (Anyway, he's a great advertiser for the products he found that he claims really do work...and this is probably closer to the truth of the matter. But you can decide for yourself. I had a customer who once told me that her particular fragrance, Chanel No 5, made her feel super sexy...and she continued, if I believe it, then it is true! (Truly case of mind over matter!)

How to Find More Perfume Samples

Tip 78: Buy women's magazines that include perfumed flaps advertising the latest fragrances on the market. This is not a true test but you can get an idea of what it smells like.

Tip 79: Check out the Perfumed Court website. They provide perfume samples that are hand poured from the original bottle of perfume that they guarantee are authentic. They repackage into a small bottle and you can order as many as you want to try out before purchasing a full bottle. They offer 'rare, vintage, discontinued, hard to find, uncommon, as well as well-known mass marketed fragrances'. Visit them at http://theperfumedcourt.com/.[10]

Tip 80: To get new mainstream releases, go to a store and ask for a sample. Robin, a regular contributor to the Now Smell This blog site for fragrances says that Nordstrom and Sephora top her 'list of the absolute best foraging grounds'. You can get manufacturer samples when available. 'They will happily decant a sample for you. [11]

Tip 81: If a company has a website, it is worth a try to write and ask for sample(s). Some of the larger companies post free sample offers online when they launch new fragrance releases. The down side to this is that it usually 4-6 weeks to receive them and they are usually packaged as liquid "bubbles" on a card or pre-moisened towelettes.[12]

A Few More Tips from My Own Experiences

Tip 82: Attend advertised perfume launches at department stores. These are fun events that usually include drawings and giveaways as part of the promotion. Plus it's great way to get free samples and try out new products.

Tip 83: Try out a friend's perfume that she either bought and does not like or it was a gift that did not work for her. It's another way to 'try before you buy'. Also, offer to buy it if your friend is hesitant to simply give it away. That way you will both be happy!

Tip 84: Thinking along this idea, host a perfume exchange party. Give guests exchange points for each new bottle or product they bring. You can also use Monopoly money or poker chips as barter. Buy small plastic or glass vials from your local beauty supply store to make samples that can be taken home.

Tip 85: I recommend that you ask for a small bag to wrap your samples and carry home to try. Saturate a few cards and be sure to write the fragrance name on it if it is not the same. Fold the cards to separate them from each other and keep from drying out.

Tip 86: (In reference to Tip 83: Just remember that just because something smells good on your girlfriend or sister does NOT mean that it will on you... it's all about that 'chemistry' thing!)

Tip 86: There are many, many sites where you can find free perfume samples and small vials for as little as one dollar! Just surf the net and see what you find!

Tip 87: Small freebie perfume vials are great to save and take on trips, especially when you fly. It is a heart break when your luggage is gone through and your fragrance bottle is removed (for whatever reason) or someone decides to 'lift' it.

Tip 88: Sign up for newsletters from perfume sites. Be one of the first to know what's new and what's hot!

Tip 89: Take your own vials or bottles and ask for a free sample or two. You can buy small sample bottles at any beauty supply stores.

Tip 90. Don't act like you are trick-or-reating though. The employees need to spread that tester bottle love and tend to frown upon freeloaders. Here's an example: "I'm having a party and want to get all the free samples I can to put into my goodie bags." Really!

A Couple More Tips from eHow

How to Get Free Perfume Samples Delivered

Tip 91: Check free sample web sites. There are a bunch of web sites like FreeSamplesDirect.com and FreebieFanatics.Blogspot.com that will give you the latest news about which perfume companies and stores are offering free perfume samples. Usually the free samples' website will direct you to the official website of the store or product so you don't have to give any information to a website you don't trust.

Tip 92: At Sephora.com, you can purchase a wide variety of makeup, beauty supplies and perfume. If you make a purchase online, Sephora's website will allow you to choose a bag of free samples, depending on how much money you spend. Best of all, you get to choose which samples you'd like to try.[13]

Lastly, A Few More of My Own Observations

Tip 93: Look online for free sample sites and sign up!

Tip 94: Look for and purchase small fragrance coffrets. These gift sets typically contain three to five small one-fourth-ounce bottles.

Tip 95: Try mixing fragrances that are more or less in the same family to create your own unique scent.

I used to know a man who layered Lagerfeld, Grey Flannel, and Green Polo. It smelled fantastic on him! It's fun to "spray and play"!

Tip 96: When mixing scents, you will want to avoid layering those that would obviously conflict. For example, a heavy woodsy, spicy scent might not go well with a strong citrus smell. On the other hand, an orange scent would layer well over something spicy.

Tip 97: Here are three things to notice if you buy at discount stores:

1. Look for clarity like a jewel tone color. However, even if the product is faded, it may still be good because light does have an effect on this.
2. Shake the bottle. If the contents bubble up but are very slow to dissipate, then it may have soured, and you should not buy it.
3. If the color is dull, the product bubbles, and you can actually see things floating around in the content, then you definitely should pass up this bargain. It has gone out of solution, and there's no telling how old it is.

Tip 98: If you really like a fragrance, but your spouse does not like that scent on you, then try to find something else that you agree on. Because if they don't like it, then it is not working for you. In other words, girls, your significant other needs to like it!

O blood type personalities are often inclined to think that they do not really care if anyone else likes their smell. But they do, and that's all that matters. I'm just saying, "You might want to rethink that."

Tip 99: It is hard to get your sexy on if your partner is turned off by your fragrance.

Tip 100: You should love, love your fragrance! If you do not like it a lot, don't wear it, no matter where it came from

Hope you enjoyed this Q&A chapter. I know it will help with your scent-sational searches for friends and family but especially for yourself!

I LOVE this quote!

When a woman is in the arms of a man she loves, in the dark of the night, the perfume she is wearing plays a very important role.

—Jean-Paul Guerlain

8

Cross-References for Fragrances

This chapter is a path to continue your searches. I've created a directory of fragrance families with lists of perfume examples for each category. You will find that I featured some of my recommendations and listed others as "Also Try" for men, women, and teens.

Keep in mind that finding a single fragrance family is not an exact science due to many other contributing bodily factors. It does guide you into a more finite area of choice.

Top Selling Perfumes for Women and Men's Fragrances

When you visit a fragrance department and notice that there seems to be more floral perfumes than other perfumes, you are correct. One reason for that, I think, is because there is such a wide variety of floral, fruity, and spicy notes that mix into endless possible combinations.

Floral variations definitely fall into the fragrance for the two largest blood types, O and A. Also, perfume houses create what sells best, and this is why perfume counters are covered with more of the floral fragrance types. The bottom line is to meet the demand of consumers and produce more of what sells.

I tend to agree that these would be considered top sellers in popular department stores.

According to Anamika S, a freelance writer for HubPages,

> Floral perfumes are those fragrances that are dominated by one or several types of flower notes. These Perfumes are mostly feminine and popular with women. Floral perfumes represent the essence of love and romance and are not only the oldest fragrances but the most popular too. Floral Perfumes can be Single Floral fragrances with one single flower scent or several blended together to produce a unique scent. Some of the popular ingredients of flower based perfumes are Roses, Orange Blossoms, Gardenias, Jasmine, Carnations, Frangipani, Lotus, Champaka, Lily of the Valley, Freesias, Aldehydes, Tuberose and other expensive natural flower oils.[1]

The following lists are top ten women and men's fragrances. Bear in mind that they will probably best satisfy the noses of the O and A blood types because they are mostly florals. Also, when a fragrance begins with fruit, the As will most likely be drawn to this scent. If citrus comes at the beginning of the notes then the Bs will want to try this. I've starred (*) the only two women's fragrances that I think may be delicate enough for the ABs.

Top Ten 2014 Fragrances for Women

1. **Si by Giorgio Armani ***
   Fragrance notes: cassis, vanilla, patchouli, freesia, rose, woods, ambroxan

2. **Velvet Orchid by Tom Ford**
   Fragrance notes: black orchid, vanilla, rum, myrrh, suede, honey, sandalwood, heliotrope, magnolia, jasmine,hyacinth, peru balsam, bergamot, orange blossom, ladanum, orange, rose

3. **Chloe by Chloe**
   Fragrance notes: rose, peony, lychee, lily of the valley, freesia, magnolia, cedar, amber

4. **Dolce by Dolce & Gabbana**
   Fragrance notes: water lily, musk, neroli, papaya flower, cashmere wood, narcissus, amaryllis

5. **Gucci Premiere by Gucci**
   Fragrance notes: bergamot, orange blossom, white flowers, musk, leather, and wood

6. **Tresor Midnight Rose by Lancome**
   Fragrance notes: raspberry, rose, cassis, vanilla, pink pepper, musk, cedar, peony, and jasmine

7. **Narciso Rodriquez for Her by Narciso Rodriguez**
   Fragrance notes: musk, rose, patchouli, sandalwood, peach, and amber

8. **Dot by Marc Jacobs**
   Fragrance notes: redberries, dragon fruit, coconut, jasmine, honeysuckle, vanilla, neroli, driftwood, and musk

9. **Bright Crystal Absolu by Versace**
    Fragrance notes: raspberry pomegranate, mognolia, peony, yuzu, lotus, musk, and amber

10. **Hypnotic Poison by Dior**
    Fragrance notes: vanilla, almond, coconut, sandalwood, orgia[2]

A great thing about this site is that they hand decanter sample bottles in three different sizes. Costs average about one dollar to three dollars. They also offer small sets of their top ten current sellers, fragrance house samples, and mini bottles of perfume. These cost from two dollars to thirty dollars and are great ways to try out what's new!

Top Ten Fragrances for Men

1. **A*Men Pure Havane by Thierry Mugler**
    Fragrance Notes: honey, tobacco, vanilla, cacao, patchouli, amber, styrax, and labdamum

2. **Armani Code Ultimate by Giorgio Armani**
    Fragrance Notes: grapefruit, mandarin, star anise, cedar, cypress, olive blossom, heliotrope, guaiac wood, tonka bean, and vanilla

3. **The One by Dolce & Gabanna**
    Fragrance Notes: tobacco, amber, ginger, grapefruit, orange blossom, cardamom, coriander, cedar, and basil

4. **Polo Red by Ralph Lauren**
    Fragrance Notes: cranberry, grapefruit, amber, coffee, woods, saffron, lemon, and sage

5. **Gucci Pour Homme II by Gucci**
   Fragrance Notes: black tea, cinnamon, violet leaf, tobacco, pimento, myrrh, bergamot, musk, and olive tree

6. **Prada Luna Rosa by Prada**
   Fragrance Notes: lavender, orange, mint, sage, ambrette, and ambroxan

7. **Legend by MontBlanc**
   Fragrance Notes: pineapple, red apple, lavender, dried fruits, bergamot, tonka bean, geranium, oakmoss, sandalwood, lemon verbena, rose, and coumarin

8. **Versace Pour Homme by Versace**
   Fragrance Notes: lemon, neroli, bergamot, tonka bean, hyacinth, rose, sage, musk, cedar, geranium, and amber

9. **Fahrenheit by Dior**
   Fragrance Notes: leather, violet leaf, vetiver, nutmeg, musk, cedar, lavender, orange, honeysuckle, sandalwood, amber, chamomile, tonka bean, patchouli, jasmine, carnation, hawthorn, lemon, bergamot, and lily of the valley

10. **Noir by Tom Ford**
    Fragrance Notes: patchouli, amber, vanilla, iris, violet, civet, rose, opoponax, vetiver, bergamot, pepper, sage, geranium, pink pepper, caraway, verbena, nutmeg, leather, benzoin, and styrax[3]

Sephora's Top Ten Best Sellers for Women and Men

WOMEN: **Flowerbomb** by Viktor & Rolf; **Stella** by Stella McCartney; **J'adore** by Dior; **Chloe** by Chloe; **Acqua di Gioia** by Giorgio Armani; **Light Blue** by Dolce & Gabanna; **Tory Burch** by Tory Burch; **Nirvana Black** by Elizabethand James; **Amazing Grace** by Philosophy; **Daisy** by Marc Jacobs; **Black Orchid** by Tom Ford[4]

MEN: **Acqua Di Gio** by Giorgio Armani; **Un Jardin sur le Nil** by Hermes; **L'Homme** by Yves St. Laurent; **Spicebomb** by Viktor & Rolph; **Terre d'Hermes** by Hermes; **Pour Homme** by Versace; **1 Million** by Paco Rabanne, **Dior Homme** by Dior; **Orange Sanguine** by Atlier; **The One** by Dolce & Gabanna[5]

Fragrance References to Families

My go-to person has always been Michael Edwards throughout my searches and the information I decided to keep and share

This chapter includes beautiful commentaries about each individual fragrance family. I have listed perfumes that fit into these families under "Recommendations" and others under "Also Try." As I tried to place them into appropriate subcategories, my search indicated that this was definitely open to conjecture!

I do not pretend to be a professional in the world of fragrance. The perfumes I have recommended are mostly the very small percentile that I have experienced, and you would find them at any shopping mall. I recently read that there are over twenty thousand fragrances in the world today. Wow!

Think about the smells you like and look for key words like floral, woodsy, spicy, vanilla, fruity, soft, bold, etc., and make a shopping list for new fun fragrance searches! Take a friend to the mall or visit or start your own "perfume swap meet." Search the Internet for the families that include notes that you love (for example, vanilla, freesia, or grapefruit). You can also search online for related samples that are free or that can be purchased for a nominal fee. Think of this exploration as a lifelong adventure for scent-sational searches!

Floral Family

- Soft Floral

   "The marriage of sparkling aldehydes and delicate flowers creates a family of soft, often powdery, abstract florals.

   Aldehydes are found naturally in rose and citrus oils, but in such minute amounts that they have to be recreated in the laboratory. Their natural scent is not pleasant: some have a sharp, metallic fragrance, others the burnt, waxy aroma of a just snuffed candle. Add them to flowers, however, and their subtle magic makes the blossoms sing. Their soprano notes are muted by the powdery accents of iris and vanilla to create a fragrance that is both soft and flowery."[6]

Recommendations:

1. Cashmere Mist by Donna Karan: This Mother's Day gift favorite is intensely feminine. It opens with lovely blends of lily of the valley, suede, bergamot, ylang-ylang, and jasmine. It also hints of sandalwood, orris, amber, vanilla, cedarwood, patchuouli, and musk.

2. Love by Coach: Desirable and chic. This modern collection of notes includes mandarin, dewberry, freesia, violet leaves, gardenia, jasmine, magnolia, patchouli, sandalwood, musk, vanilla, and caramel.
3. Flash by Jimmy Choo: "Anticipation. Excitement. The cool rush of power embodies the thrill of dressing up with a fresh, sparkline introduction of pink pepper, tangerine and strawberry. Heart notes of strong, exotic white flowers (tuberose, jasmine, white lily, heliotrope) and base of white powdery woods leaves a lasting impression, both seductive and sensual."[7]

Also Try:
BCBG Max Azria Bon Chic by Max Azria
N°5 Eau Premiere by Chanel
Sensuous Nude by Estée Lauder

• Floral
"Florals remain the most popular fragrance family. Their repertoire is vast, ranging from concertos on the theme of a single floral note to mighty symphonies of heady mixed bouquets.

Headspace technology has given perfumers an avalanche of exciting new floral notes: it allows them to identify and clone the scent of blooms from which no oil can be extracted by traditional methods. Each year, unusual new notes are found, revitalising the traditional floral theme."[8]

Recommendations:

1. Chanel N°5 for Women
   "In 1921, Coco Chanel asked perfumer Ernest Beaux to create something that "smells like woman." The resulting elixir would become the world's most iconic fragrance, beloved by legions of women including Marilyn Monroe, who famously stated she wore nothing else to bed. A blend of luxurious florals and warm base notes, including ylang-ylang, rose, iris, neroli and vanilla, No. 5 is an elegant, womanly scent that transitions well from day to nighttime wear."[9]

2. Lovestruck Floral Rush by Vera Wang
   "This fragrance possesses a blend of champagne accord, apricot blossom, pink passion flower, cashmere woods, sheer musk, pink pepper, marigold, freesia and white amber."[10]

3. Trésor by Lancome for Women
   "Tresor is a deeply romantic fragrance. Lush and unabashedly floral, with pretty top notes of lilac and apricot, this is an intensely feminine perfume that charms more than it seduces. Wear it with confidence on a first date, or to a special dinner with your long-term love."[11]

Also Try:
Gucci Rush by Gucci
L'Air du Temps by Nina Ricci;
Tuberose Gardenia by Estée Lauder

- Floral Oriental
  "The marriage of sparkling aldehydes and delicate flowers creates a family of soft, often powdery, abstract florals.

  Soft, spicy orange flower notes meld with piquant aldehydes and sweet spices to create the heart of a Floral Oriental fragrance. Born in the 1900s, Floral Orientals came back to life again in the 1970s. In the past decade, lively, fruity interpretations dominated the Floral Oriental category, but recent fragrances have developed a more subtle, muted personality."[12]

Recommendations:

1. Alien by Thierry Mugler
   "Alien combines notes of vanilla, amber, and orange blossom with a hint of the woods to create a spicy, oriental scent that is not overpowering. Introduced in 2005, it is perfect for casual outings, such as running errands or a lunch date with friends. Spritz Alien behind your ears before heading out the door to provide an extra boost of confidence as you turn heads wherever you go."[13]

2. Chloe by Karl Lagerfield for Women
   "Chloe was created by Karl Lagerfeld when he helmed the fashion house of Chloe (now run by Stella McCartney). Like Lagerfeld's clientele, which included Maria Callas and Jaqueline Kennedy-Onassis, this fragrance is rich, romantic and powerful. Jasmine and honeysuckle are layered over spices and woods, to create a fragrance that is boldly feminine."[14]

Also Try:
Cashmere Mist by Donna Karan
Eternity by Calvin Klein
The One by Dolce & Gabbana.

Oriental Family

*   Soft Oriental
    "Incense adds sensual overtones to fragrant flowers, spices and amber to create a softer style of Oriental.

    The base notes of a modern Soft Oriental are not as sweet or as heavy as a true Oriental and the result—a mélange of flowers and spices—is distinctly softer."[15]

Recommendations:
1. Boucheron for women
    "The delicate scent is introduced by lively green and fruity top notes, then develops into an intense heart of sensual florals. Underscoring the arrangement are warm, woody background notes, sensual and long-lasting. Top Notes Include: tangerine, bitter orange, apricot. Heart Notes: orange blossom, tuberose, ylang-ylang, jasmine, narcissus. Base Notes: sandalwood, amber, vanilla, tonka bean."[16]
2. Miracle by Lancome
    "This feminine fragrance is both modern and sophisticated. Top notes sparkle with freesia and lychee. The power of spice breaks through the middle notes lighting the fragrance with ginger and pepper. The heart reveals sensual notes of jasmine and magnolia."[17]

3. Obsession Cologne for Men by Calvin Klein
   "A casual but distinctive daytime scent for men is
   a spicy, moderate fragrance that balances its citrus notes with musky undertones. Also dominant
   notes of spice and mandarin with low tones of
   musk, amber and sandalwood. This appealing and
   resonant fragrance is the perfect choice for a broad
   variety of daytime events."[18]

   Also Try:
   Allure by Chanel (masculine and feminine).

• Oriental
   "Sensual, often heavy, blends of oriental resins,
   opulent flowers, sweet vanilla and musks are
   introduced by refreshing citrus, green or fruity
   top notes.
   The new 'sheer' Orientals gained some ground
   in the late 1990s, but the appeal of the full-bodied,
   take-no-prisoners Orientals endures. Orientals are
   the exotic queens of perfumery."[19]

Recommendations:
1. Angel by Thierry Mugler
   "Created in 1992, Angel perfume is a chocolate
   vanilla oriental, woody fragrance. Angel perfume is
   a feminine scent that possesses a blend of vanilla,
   sandalwood, and patchouli. Accompanied by fruity
   notes of fresh citrus, melons, peaches, and plums."[20]
2. Amarige by Givenchy
   "Is classified as a sharp, oriental, floral fragrance.
   This feminine scent possesses a blend of violet,
   mimosa, soft sweet spices, and orange flowers.

Accompanied by fruity notes of fresh citrus, melons, peaches, and plums."[21]

3. Shalimar by Guerlain Fragrances
"Shalimar is a fragrance to excite and express desire. She who dares to wear it, is asserting her femininity and ultra sensuality. Surrender to the scents of lemon, bergamot, jasmine, May rose, iris, incense, opoponax, tonka bean, and vanilla."[22]

Also Try:
Coco by Chanel
H.O.T. Always by Bond No. 9
Weekend by Burberry.

• Woody Oriental
"The liaison of rich Oriental notes and the potent scents of patchouli and sandalwood produced some of the most original perfumes of the 1990s.

This family emphasizes the woody character of Floral Orientals. The key difference is that their flowers and spices play second string to the dominant sandalwood and/or patchouli notes. The Oriental influence is more noticeable, too, and balances the deep wood notes."[23]

Recommendations:
1. Gucci Guilty Black
Bold and spicy, Gucci's newest scent features notes of lavender, coriander, orange, and patchouli.
2. CK One Shock for Him by Calvin Klein
This masculine oriental blends mandarin, cucumber, pepper, cardamom, tobacco, musk, and patchouli.

3. Angel B Men by Thierry Mugler
    A casual intoxicating scent of citrus, vanilla musk,
    and cedar wood that creates a woody and spicy fra-
    grance.

    Men/Also Try:
    Bvlgari BLV pour Homme
    Allure Homme Sport by Chanel
    Rush for Men by Gucci

    Women/Also Try:
    Gold Rose 2012 by Michael Kors
    Harrods Jubilee 2012 by Bond No. 9
    Miroir de Voluptes by Thierry Mugler
    Women can try Gold Rose 2012 by Michael Kors,
    Harrods Jubilee 2012 by Bond No. 9, and Miroir
    de Voluptes by Thierry Mugler.

This woody notes section appeals mostly to men;
however, I found that some women with O and B blood
types quite often enjoy fragrances found on the men's
counters. The Bs like bolder crisp scents, and Os like the
woodsy fragrances. I particularly like The One by Dolce &
Gabanna and enjoy the men's version for evening and the
women's for day.

Woody Notes

*   Classic Woods
        "Lately, perfumers have rediscovered woody
    notes in a big way, so it makes sense to distinguish
    them from the Chypre or Mossy Woods fragrances.
        Classic woody scents are dominated by harmonies
    of cedar, patchouli, pine, sandalwood and vetiver but

a new palette of exotic wood notes–often cloned from headspace technology–has stimulated greater creativity in this neglected fragrance category."[24]

Recommendations:

1. Acqua di Gio by Giorgio Armani
   "Introduced in 1997 and often touted as today's No. 1 men's fragrance. "It has the bright fresh scent of citrus smoothly blended with a rosemary spiciness and jasmine with a wood base. The woody scent evokes the freedom of the outdoors with the slightly bitter citrus tone providing the illusion of fresh breezes in tropical climates."[25]

2. L'Homme by Yves Saint Laurent
   "A very masculine scent that's balanced by a spicy, moderate tone, perfect for the man who has an appreciation for subtlety and contemporary culture. This casual fragrance is punctuated by notes of citron, white pepper, Virginia cedar, vetiver, ginger and basil flower. For the sophisticated man on the go, a great complement to casual occasions."[26]

3. Wild Fig by Joe Malone
   "Inspired by breakfast in Tuscany the moment of breaking open juicy figs, fresh from the tree. This delicious fragrance of figs and cassis is entwined with notes of hyacinth and cedarwood that envelopes the wearer in the warmth of the Mediterranean."[27]

Men/Also Try:
Cuba Gold, Woods by Abercrombie & Fitch
Blanc by Lacoste
London by Jo Malone

Men can also try Cuba Gold, Woods by Abercrombie & Fitch, Blanc by Lacoste, London by Jo Malone, and Kanon Norwegian Wood.

- Dry Woods
  "The Dry Woods family is often called Leather, after the dry, smoky scent of Russian leather.

  Fresh citrus notes play an important role in most Dry Woods fragrances, lightening the deep, almost animalic heart notes. A mossy-woody fragrance takes on a drier character with the addition of cedar, tobacco and burnt wood notes."[28]

Recommendations:

1. Cordovan by Banana Republic
   "This casual fragrance perfectly combines the scents of leafy green fig, white juniper berries, and vetiver root with subtle notes of vintage leather, iced lavender and woody orris. The resulting fragrance is a very masculine blend that's perfect for everyday use."[29]

2. Tuscan Leather by Tom Ford
   "A chypre blend of notes brings a raw yet reserved sensuality to this classic leather scent. Saffron, raspberry and thyme open to olibanum and night-blooming jasmine. Leather, black suede and amber wood add an intricate richness."[30]

3. Spicebomb by Vikto and Rolf
   "This explosive cocktail of virility transforms you into a powerful, intense and daring man. Top notes: bergamot, grapefruit, pink pepper, elemi. Middle: cinnamon, chili pepper, saffron. Base: leather, vetiver, tobacco."[31]

Also Try:
Only the Brave by Diesel
Gucci Guilty Black
Vintage by John Varvatos

• Mossy Woods
"Perfumers call these forest notes of oakmoss, amber and citrus Chypre fragrances.

The family takes its name from the first significant mossy-woody fragrance, Chypre de Coty, created by François Coty in 1917. Chypre is the French name for the island of Cyprus, birthplace of Venus, the legendary goddess of love. From Cyprus, too, comes the oakmoss that is at the heart of all fragrances."[32]

Recommendations:
1. Ferrari Black by Ferrari
   This is a perfect fragrance for casual outings. It mixes crisp woodsy and mossy notes to add a touch of excitement to your day.
2. Nautica Voyage by Nautica.
   Makes casual days smooth sailing with notes of amber, mimosa, apple, cedar, and musk.

Men/Also Try:
Armani ManiaAramisHugo

• Aromatic Fougere
"This is the universal fragrance family, with sexy cool-warm notes of citrus and lavender, sweet spices and oriental woods. It takes its name from a fragrance long since discontinued: Fougère Royale, introduced by Houbigant in 1882. Men grew up

on Fougères. Most of the key men's fragrances developed since the mid-1960s have come from this family; their zesty, masculine character makes men feel comfortable. Most women, too, find the blend of Fresh, Floral, Oriental and Woody notes appealing. It is a winning combination."[33]

Recommendations:

1. Acqua di Gio by Giorgio Armani
   This contains the following fragrance notes: lavender, juniper, and cumin. It is accented with ylang-ylang, sandalwood, and amber.
2. Bvlgari Man
   This distinctive contemporary fragrance is both elegant and sophisticated. Opening notes include white pear and bergamot with a heart of pure cashmere wood and vetiver. It dries down on tonka bean and musk.
3. Dolce & Gabbana
   This is another sophisticated scent that has been a great evening choice for over twenty-five years. Its signature combines lavender and citrus notes of orange and lemon with base aromas of cedar, tobacco, and sage.
   Men/Also Try:
   Euphoria by Calvin Klein
   Guess Suede
   Kenneth Cole Black

Fresh Notes

- Fruity
  "Peaches and pears, apples and plums. A twist of tropical fruits. Essences of strawberry, raspberry and berries of all hues. Add a splash of flowers to create a family of fruity cocktails that smell delicious."[34]

Recommendations:

1. Angel by Thierry Mugler
   This intriguing fragrance, created in 1992, was the first gourmand fragrance and first blue fragrance, and it is featured in a beautiful refillable star. Perfect for your daytime adventures, its delicious notes include vanilla, tropical fruits, and caramel with touches of patchouli and bergamot.
2. Miss Dior Cherie by Christian Dior for Women. This modern fragrance is perfect for chic teens while it reflects the timeless elegance of Dior. Its youthful scent blends notes of green tangerine, violet, and pink jasmine that mingle with soft patchouli, sweet strawberry, and caramelized popcorn.

   Girls/Also Try:
   A Is for ALDO Red by ALDO
   Skulls & Roses for Her by Ed Hardy
   Love Hope Denim by True Religion.

- Green
  "Green fragrances capture the sharp scent of fresh-cut grass and violet leaves.
       Despite the outdoors imagery, the impact of the classic resinous galbanum accord is so potent that

many green fragrances have a formal rather than sporty personality. In recent years, a palette of softer, lighter green notes has given this fragrance family fresh appeal."[35]

Recommendations:

1. N°19 by Chanel

    "This luminous re-imagining of Coco Chanel's signature scent—named N°19 in honor of her birth date, August 19, 1883—reveals a bold fragrance with a daring combination of crisp green notes and powdery iris."[36]

2. Lauren by Ralph Lauren.

    These green florals are perfect for women who like a crisp scent, and it is great for day or informal evening events. Carnations, violets, and roses—the rare wood spices—complete the fragrance.

3. Acqua di Gioia by the designer house of Giorgio Armani.

    This was created for the woman who is strong, dignified, and free-spirited. Its composition pushes the limit between crushed mint and lemon and the floral heart of aquatic jasmine and peony. It closes in a base of cedar and yellow sugar.

Also Try:

Lauren by Ralph Lauren and Beautiful by Estée Lauder.

- Water

    "Redolent of the scent of soft sea breezes, the marine notes were created in 1990. The early water notes captured the ozonic aroma of wet air after a thunderstorm. Today, the water notes are more often used as an accent to enliven florals, orientals and woody fragrances."[37]

Recommendations:

1. Aqua di Gio for Women by Giorgio Armani. "This aquatic floral is a fresh take on the category combines fresh floral scents with marine and fruity notes, over a musky base. Wear this clean, feminine fragrance when you need a mood-booster."[38]

2. He Wood Ocean Wet Wood by DSQUARED2. "Subtly blends ocean, wet, and wood accords to create a masculine fragrance inspired by nature. It features ocean accords of artemisia and ambergris, wet accords of violet and musk, and wood accords of patchouli and tonka bean that result in a light fragrance."[39]

Also Try:
Desire Blue by Alfred Dunhill
Eternity Aqua by Calvin Klein
Pure by Boss

• Citrus
"From the zest of lemons, mandarins, bergamot, oranges and grapefruit come the citrus oils that lend these fragrances their distinctive, tangy aroma. Floral, spicy and woody notes transformed the light, refreshing eaux de cologne into real fragrances. A new generation of musk and tea accents adds an interesting dimension to the oldest fragrance family."[40]

Feminine Recommendations:

1. CK One by Calvin Klein

   "One of the first successful unisex fragrances, CK One awakens the senses with notes of papaya, pineapple, lemon and floral notes, over a base accord of green tea. A refreshing, clean scent that's light enough to wear to breakfast." [41]

2. Close for Women by Gap.

   This clean fresh scent is perfect for any daytime date. Salty citrus layers over a spicy musky base.

3. Clinique Happy for Women

   Happy is a Clinique signature scent that blends the freshness of oranges and pink grapefruit with crisp florals for an airy feminine fragrance. It is a great pick-you-upper when a lift of spirit is needed.

Masculine Recommendations:
Armani Code Sport
Pony Blue 1 by Polo
Sunset Voyage by Nautica

Teen Fragrances

The next scents are perfect for young women but also for the young at heart who simply want a lighter fragrance. I've selected them based on personality types.

For Girls:

1. Daisy Eau So Fresh by Marc Jacobs.

   This fruity floral is a good choice for the creative outgoing girl. Blends of ruby red grapefruit, raspberry, pear, and plum are centered with wild rose and jasmine, and finally, it gives off a cedar edge.

2. Hippie Chic by True Religion.

   Recommended for the true romantic, this fragrance tempts with the fruits of pomegranate, apple, and raspberry. Its flowers, jasmine and hibiscus, dry down to sheer woods and musk.

3. True Religion for Women.

   This is recommended for the delicate chemistries of those who are sensitive to flowers. It blends sparkling fruits with pear blossoms and warm wood notes to create soft, sheer loveliness.

Ralph Lauren's Big Pony Collection

To target the young adult market, Ralph Lauren's Big Pony collections were launched. The "Axe generation" (male) and what I fondly refer to as the (female) "bubblegum brigade" were given distinctive fresh fragrances that spoke to their youth. They can be worn by anybody who wants a nice, light day fragrance. In my opinion, there is a scent for each blood type (BT).

Feminine:

- Big Pony #1: The Blue is a sporty citrus and floral blend of grapefruit and blue lotus. (BT B)
- Big Pony #2: The Pink is a fruity floral blend of cranberry and tonka mousse. I noticed it to be the top seller of the four families. (BT A)
- Big Pony #3: The Yellow is blend of pear and mimosa. (BT AB)
- Big Pony #4: The Purple is a floriental blend of wild cherry and amber. (BT O)

Masculine:
- Big Pony #1: The Blue is a blend of aromatic grapefruit, lime and oak. Most like the men's Blue. (BT B)
- Big Pony #2: The Red scent possesses a blend of dark chocolate and musk. Most like men's Black. (BT AB)
- Big Pony #3: The Orange is a blend of Mandarin orange and kyara wood. (Most like men's double black for BT-O.)
- Big Pony #4: The Green is a blend of ginger and mint. Most like Polo Classic (green). (BT A)

Blood Type Fragrance Lists

The following lists fragrance families by house or Design and recommends perfumes for specific blood types (BT). This sampling is intended to only give an idea of how these families will work with your blood type. One can follow up for more choices by checking the notes and finding other fragrances that include more of the same. Visit any of the sites listed at the end of the chapter for more options.

Feminine

- Florals (for BT O and A)
    Light for Casual Use: N°5 Eau Premiere by Chanel, EuphoriaCalvin Klein, Cashmere Mist by Donna Karan, Daisy Eau So Fresh by Marc Jacobs.
    Rich for Evening Use: Forbidden Euphoria by Calvin Klein, Chanel N°5, J'adore by Christian Dior, Tuberose Gardenia by Estée Lauder, and Trèsor Midnight Rose by Lancôme.

- Soft Floral (for BT A and AB)
  Burberry Body, Chance Eau Tendre by Chanel, Dolce & Gabbana Light Blue, Cashmere Mist by Donna Karan, and Daisy by Marc Jacobs.
- Oriental (for BT O, A, and B)
  In Control Curious by Britney Spears; Eternity by Calvin Klein; Allure, Coco, and Coco Mademoiselle by Chanel; The One by Dolce & Gabbana; Gucci Guilty Black.
- Fresh (for BT A and B)
  Burberry Classic and Summer, Chance Eau Fraiche by Chanel, Clinique Happy, Coach Poppy Flower, Viva La Juicy by Juicy Couture.

Fragrance Sample Databases

Filthy Fragrance.com: created to provide access to top brand fragrances at huge discounts by eliminating the middle man. Save up to 80 % on products, and get free shipping on orders over $59.00. They stand by their 100% money back guarantee with a hassle free return policy. "With prices so low, they're downright filthy".

FragranceNet.com: This is a go-to place for discounted fragrances. It's a great site for women's and men's products. It has alphabetized drop-down lists to find perfumes by name. It also has really good descriptions that includes the notes.

Fragrancesoftheworld.info: This site allows you to sort, cross-reference, and discover accurate information on more than twelve thousand selective, niche, mass, and direct retail fragrances.

FreebieFanatics.blogspot.com
FreeSamplesDirect.com

My Perfume Samples: myperfumesamples.com. This company hand-pours samples for both women's and men's fragrances and three sizes for as low as ninety-nine cents. They also specialize in mini bottles priced up to twenty dollars that are perfect for travel.

Parfums Raffy: parfumsraffy.com/perfume-samples. This is a great site! Search men's and women's perfumes alphabetically. The site also offers free sample. They also have women's colognes listed by manufacturer in the drop-down list at the top right of every page. A comprehensive list of perfume manufacturers can be found on their designer fragrances page.

The Perfumed Court: theperfumedcourt.com. They specialize in perfume samples and hand poured decants from the original bottle of fragrance. Customer does not receive licensed products.

Thierry Mugler: muglerstoreusa.com: You can enjoy free shipping with any order and free Thierry Mugler samples.

yourfragrancecollection.com

9

Final Thoughts

"Why?" This is always my big question.

My desire to learn more began at a very young age. I was one of those little kids who always asked "Why?" When my questions exhausted my mom's patience, she would serve me with her standard "Because I said so," but that usually only dampened my curiosity. I have always loved learning, discovering new things, and working out any kind of puzzle.

When I actually began working on *Scent-sational Searches*, I was only looking for answers to satisfy *my* curiosity about fragrance choices. I searched the Internet and located relative pieces about the world of perfumery, but I could not find the answer to my one big question: *"Why does perfume smell different on people?"*

It was like trying to work a gigantic jigsaw puzzle that to date has not been completely solved. I've decided that the answer has no absolutes as in math equations. It is my belief, however, that there are major factors that have been proven to determine our biological "being-ness" and map our characteristics.

A commonality regarding fragrances is that we have all had "scent-sational" moments in our lives that can be related to our sense of smell. Think back to your early formative years and about smells or tastes that stand out in your mind's eye. These memories can evoke either good or bad recollections that have already scented your life.

On a grander scale

We are all part of God's universal creation. I recently heard an astrophysicist on a Georgia public TV show say that humans all "have intricate pieces of star dust in their deepest inner level of creation." Think of your biological self as pure energy that comes together in cells of flesh and blood. These energy forces are woven together by unseen magnetic waves that align into what we know as genetics.

While searching more deeply, I learned that DNA factors copy and transfer into our genetic pool. This caused me to ponder whether or not memories are also carried forward. I cannot help but wonder how much of our birth is predisposed with specific personality, likes, and dislikes because of ancestral memories. How else can one explain a child prodigy? How much more do we inherit beyond our physical characteristics?

A recently published study from Rockefeller University, found *that the human nose can detect at least one trillion smells.* Researchers tested people's sense of smell by using different mixtures of odor molecules. Prior to this, scientists thought that only about ten thousand different smells could be detected.[1]

I think this awareness will open the door for a huge wave of new fragrance combinations. If I were a researcher helping to create new fragrances, I would definitely think about a new perspective to please individual olfactory nerves and their cranial connection. *This would be how one actually feels and thinks about something they smell or taste, especially perfumes!*

Sorting out factors that match blood/personality types to senses of smell and taste could be a giant step in the process of elimination of what will work for specific body chemistries. For example, my theory points out that Os love woodsy, strong florals that may lean toward spicy notes; however, they do not usually enjoy sharp citrus scents in their mix.

To put this into another perspective, you probably would not enjoy caviar that was covered with peanut butter. What about chocolate pudding on top of Carolina barbequed ribs? I think not! They simply would not go together. Also, it would be an expensive endeavor to satisfy the demand of the few potential customers who might really enjoy this weird combo.

Perfumers want to target masses, which is why most fragrances please the O and A blood types. Remember, they make up over 80 percent of the blood population.

Another question is, "Why do I like the way a fragrance smells but it changes when I wear it?" For example, I really love the smell of two of Dolce & Gabanna fragrances. The One is fabulous on me, but Light Blue changes to something akin to bug spray! And I've heard that same comment from more than a few women.

I've also heard many salespeople make ridiculous statements regarding perfumes like "It's a favorite of mine that I also wear myself. I know you'll like it too." Maybe, maybe not. *Keep in mind: it's not about them!*

Here's another sales approach that makes me want to roll my eyes: "This is the latest perfume from (celebrity name). Everybody wants this. It's so popular." *This is definitely not a good reason to purchase anything.*

A helpful person might ask about who you are "gifting" as well as about your favorite fragrances and if there's anything in particular that you do not like (for example, vanilla, patchouli or jasmine). When someone takes a few minutes to get to know you, they can guide you to something new in the same family but also help you steer clear of notes that you may find offensive.

How great would it be in the future if fragrances could be identified for blood type/personality by a small code printed on the perfume box? For example, O/A, you could simply look for this small code to recognize a probable O blood type/A personality perfume match.

How easy would that be? It might not be a perfect match, but at least you would be in the right family and pass over perfumes that most likely are not good personal choices.

Such a small indicator or code could help prevent an unhappy experience of searching counters for fragrance only to come up empty-handed. Or even worse, you could purchase a fragrance that just does not work for the receiver or the significant other really does not like the way it smells.

This is an awkward mistake that can also be costly if not exchanged.

Until future research gives us better ways to have "scent-sational searches," here's my best tip: *follow the idea of matching blood/personality types to fragrance families.*

Scent-sational Searches gives you the tools that will empower you with a greater understanding of why some fragrances are good choices while others are not. Whether you are gifting yourself or someone else, your searches become so much easier.

Thanks for reading my book. I hope these final thoughts will spark your curiosity to discover what your "fragranista" type is. I invite you to follow my Web site and share with your friends on all your social media accounts. Join discussions and post questions and be sure to share your fave fragrances with me at deborahworley.com

Afterword by Deborah Worley
Brain Disorders

Let's Make a Difference through Pilot Clubs International

In the past I was an active member of a service organization called Pilot Club International. I worked my way up the ranks and served as club president in 1987. During my affiliation with the organization, I developed a passion for the club's fund-raising projects for brain disorders.

A few years later, I landed a position as the marketer for an assisted living/dementia facility in Hilton Head, South Carolina. There I saw firsthand the devastation of this horrific disease and had a heartfelt desire to somehow truly make a difference on the impact of brain disorders.

As I thought about marketing my book, I had the idea to reach out to my Pilot Club friends. Here was a way to get out two stories. I could sell books through their clubs and help raise funds for the treatment of brain disorders by donating a portion of my profits back to the clubs who worked with me.

Contact me at: dworley107@yahoo.com to partner with me and find out more about how we can 'make a difference' for brain disorders through Pilot Club fund raising.

To find out more about Pilot Club International, organizations in your area or how you can join, visit their web site: pilotinternational.org. Also, to read more about the Brainhealth research center in Dallas, Texas visit their website: http://www.brainhealth.utdallas.edu/index.php/research/research_topic/alzheimers

Notes

Prologue: The "Fragranista" Begins

1. Dr. Peter D'Adamo, *Eat Right for Your Type.*
2. Ozmoz.com, Encyclo
   1 Perfume Evolution
   1. Ozmoz.com, Encyclo
2. See note 1 above.
3. See note 1 above.
4. See note 1 above.
5. See note 1 above.
6. See note 1 above.
7. See note 1 above.
8. See note 1 above.
9. See note 1 above.
10. See note 1 above.
11. See note 1 above.
12. Catherine Capozzi, "Perfume Market Analysis," http://www.ehow.com/info.7743468-perfume-market-analysis.html
13. www.vintageadbrowser.com/perfume-ads

2 The Buzz about Blood

1. "All about Blood Type History," LisaShea.com/lisabase/biology/art14433.html
2. Michael Schirber, "The Chemistry of Life: The Human Body", html LiveScience.com. http://www.livescience.com/3505-chemistry-life-human-body.
3. Blood Type Distribution by Country: ABO and Rh Distribution by Country," http://wikipedia.org/wiki/Blood_type_distribution_by_country
4. Japanese Culture 101: Personality by Blood Type," The Great Greek Manual, (1 February 2007): http://thegreatgreekmanual.com/blog/japanese-culture-101-personality-personality-by-blood-type
5. Ruth Evans, *"Japan and blood types: Does it determine personality?"* 4 November 2012: http://www.bbc.com/news/magazine-20170787.
6. http://en.wikipedia.org./wiki/Blood-types-in-Japanese-culture#Takeji-Furukawa
7. Natalie Josep, *"Can Blood Type Determine Your Personality,"* (December 2008): http:www.divinecaroline.com/self/horoscopes/can-blood-type-determine-your-personality.
8. See note 4

3 Four Basic Fragrance Families

1. "Fragrance Families," http://theperfumedcourt.com/fragrance_families.aspx.
2. See note 1 above.

4 Get to Know the Fragrance Wheel and Fragranista Chart

1. www.fragrancesoftheworld/michaeledwards
2. Http://anamikas.hubpages.com/hub/Top-10-FloralPerfumes-for-Women. (February 2, 2015)
3. "Perfumery," Wikipedia:

5 Putting It All Together

1. "How to Choose the Right Perfume for Your Body Chemistry," Beauty and the Bath (August 24, 2012): http://www.beauty-and-the-bath.com/How-To-Choose-The-Right-Perfume-For-Your-Body-Chemistry.html.
2. Lane Madison, "Foods That Affect Pheromones," eHow.com: http://www.ehow.com/facts_5619564_foods-affect-pheromones.html.
3. youbeauty.com/skin/galleries/sexy-scents-that-are-proven-to-seduce.
4. Perfume," Wikipedia:
5. http://www.aworldofplenty.com/EOFODifferences.html. Differences Among Strengths
6. How to Know When Not to Wear Perfume," eHow.com: http://www.ehow.com/how_2034430_wear-perfume.html#ixzz284U6xsDa
7. http://beauty.about.com/od/fragramc1/a/perfume-ingredients-glossary.htm

6 Bios of My Fave Perfumers

1. Coco Chanel," Biography.com. (2012):www.biography.com/people/coco-chanel.
2. "Estée Lauder," Biography.com :

3. www.fashionmodeldirectory.com/designers/ thierry-mugler

4. www.cirquedusoleil.com/zumanity/resources/creators/ thierry-mugler.

5. www.shiseido.co.jp/releimg/1790-e.pdf.

6. www.marieclaire.co.uk/fashion/thierry-mugler-to-design-beyonce-tour

7. kits/shows/zumanity/resources/creators/thierry-mugler.aspx

8. www.Sephora

9. http://www.fragrancesoftheworld.com/About-MichaelEdwards.aspx.

7 One Hundred Fragrance Tips: Q&A

1. "Top 100 Perfume Questions," Michael Edwards: http://www.fragrancesoftheworld.com/top-100questions.aspx.

2. "How to Wear Perfume," eHow.com: http://www.ehow.com/how_2126815_wear-perfume.html.

3. Valerie Kalfrin, "How to Make Perfume Last Longer," eHow.com: http://www.ehow.com/how_4798697_perfume-last-longer.html.

4. "How to Make Perfumes Last on Your Skin," eHow.com: http://www.ehow.com/how_2034360_make-perfume-last.html.

5. Michael Stone, *Celebrities Move Beyond Fragrance to Tap Other Senses Within Health & Beauty*, Forbes (December 07, 2012):

6. Karl Gramer, "Human Pheromones and Sexual Attraction," *European Journal of Obstetrics and Gynecology and Reproductive Biology* 118 (2005):

7. Warren S. T. Hays, "Human pheromones: have they been demonstrated?" *Behavioral Ecological Sociobiology* 54 (2): 98–97 (2003): doi:10.1007/s00265–003–0613–4.
8. KeVerne EB, "The Vomeronasal Organ," Science 286 (540): 716–720 (1999):
9. www.truth-about-pheromens.com
10. http://the perfumedcourt.com/
11. http://ww.nstperfume.com/2007/04/09/perfumists-tip-how-to-get-fragrance-samples-free-or-otherwise/
12. See note 11.
13. Megan Smith, "How to Get Free Perfume Samples Delivered," eHow.com: http://www.ehow.com/how_4452218_get-free-perfume-samples-delivered.html.

8 Cross-References for Fragrances

1. Anamika S., "Top 10 Floral Perfumes for Women," HubPages, February 2, 1015 http://anamikas.hubpages.com/hub/Top-10-Floral-Perfumes-for-Women
2. http://www.myperfumesamples.com/mps/top-10-fragrances-of-2014-for-women.
3. See note 2.
4. http://www.sephora.com/womens-fragrance.
5. http://www.sephora.com/mens-fragrance.
6. http://www.fragrancesoftheworld.com/external/wheel/index.html
7. http://filthyfragrance.com/Flash-3.4-oz-EDP-for-women
8. See note 6.

9. http://beauty.about/od/fragrance1/p/Splurge-Or-Steal-Perfumes.html.

10. http://www.perfumania.com/shop/womens/loves-truck-floral-rush-for-women-by-vera-wang-eau-de-parfum-spray_196606.1.html.

11. http:// http://beauty.about/od/fragrance1/tp/floral-perfumes.htm.

12. See Note 6

13. http://www.fragrancenet.com/perfume/thierry-mugler/alien/eau-de-parfum#!203293.

14. See note 11.

15. See note 6.

16. http://www.perfumania.com/shop/womens/boucheron-for-women-by-boucheron-eau-de-toilette-spray_1000900.1.html.

17. http://radiantsecrets.wordpress.com/2014/09/09/10-great-feminine-perfumes/.

18. See note 13.

19. See Note 6.

20. http://www.amazon.com/ANGEL-Thierry-Mugler-Perfume PARFUM/dp/B004V41VT0

21. http://www.perfumania.com/shop/womens/amarige-for-women-by-givenchy-eau-de-toilette-spray_999806.1.html.

22. http://www.polyvore.com/guerlain_perfume/shop?query=guerlain+perfume

23. See Note 6.

24. See Note 6.

25. http://www.fragrancenet.com/cologne/giorgio-armani/acqua-di-gio

26. http://www.fragrancenet.com/cologne/yves-saint-laurent/lhomme-yves-saint-laurent

27. http://www1.bloomingdales.com/shop/product/
jo-malone-wild-fig-cassis-collection
28. See Note 6.
29. http://orvora.com/banana-republic-cordovan-
cologne-by-banana-republic-2048.html.
30. http://www.parisgallery.com/product.php?Paris-
Gallery-TOM+FORD-TOM+FORD+
Tuscan+Leather
31. http://www.publicitymag.com/men-fine-
cologne-2014/.
32. See Note 6.
33. See Note 6.
34. See Note 6.
35. See Note 6.
36. http://shop.nordstrom.com/s/chanel-n19-po-
udre-eau-de-parfum-spray/3209704
37. See Note 6.
38. http://beauty.about.com/od/fragranc1/tp/floral-
perfumes.htm.
39. http://www.fragrancenet.com/cologne/dsquared2/
he-wood-ocean-wet-wood/edt
40. See Note 6.
41. http://beauty.about.com/od/fragranc1/tp/best-
citrus-perfumes-and-fragrances.htm

9: Final Thoughts

1. http://www.everydayhealth.com/news/incredi-
ble-facts-about-your-sense-smell/

Photos and Images

Chapter 1

Photo 1. 1920s Vintage ad
Photo 2. 1920s Vintage ad
Photo 3. 1930s Vintage ad
Photo 4. 1940s Vintage ad
Photo 5. 1940s Vintage ad
Photo 6. 1950s Vintage ad
Photo 7. 1970s Vintage ad
Photo 8. 1970s Vintage ad

Chapter 2
Image 8. Japanese test "Ketsueki-gata"

Chapter 3
1. Fairy bee

Chapter 6
1. Coco Chanel
2. Estee Lauder
3. Thierry Mugler
4. Michael Edwards